A WOMAN'S GUIDE TO HEART ATTACK RECOVERY

How to Survive, Thrive, and Protect Your Heart

A WOMAN'S GUIDE TO HEART ATTACK RECOVERY

How to Survive, Thrive, and Protect Your Heart

HARVEY M. KRAMER, M.D.,
AND CHARLOTTE LIBOV

M. EVANS
Lanham • New York • Boulder • Toronto • Plymouth, UK

Published by M. Evans
An imprint of The Rowman & Littlefield Publishing Group, Inc.
4501 Forbes Boulevard, Suite 200, Lanham, Maryland 20706

Estover Road
Plymouth PL6 7PY
United Kingdom

Distributed by NATIONAL BOOK NETWORK

Library of Congress Cataloging-in-Publication Data
Kramer, Harvey M., 1952–
  A woman's guide to heart attack recovery : how to survive, thrive, and protect
your heart / Harvey M. Kramer and Charlotte Libov.
     p. cm.
  ISBN-13: 978-1-59077-130-3 (pbk. : alk. paper)
  ISBN-10: 1-59077-130-3 (pbk. : alk. paper)
  1. Heart diseases in women—Popular works. 2. Myocardial infarction—Popular
works. 3. Women—Health and hygiene—Popular works. I. Libov, Charlotte.
II. Title.
  RC672.K74 2007
  616.1'20082—dc22   2006036432

∞™ The paper used in this publication meets the minimum requirements
of American National Standard for Information Services—Permanence of
Paper for Printed Library Materials, ANSI/NISO Z39, 48–1992.

I would like to thank my lovely wife, Suzanne, for her encouragement, support and tolerance of this multiyear project. I also wish to thank my children, Blake, Kendall, and Grayson, for affording me the time to work on this book. The inspiration from my many wonderful women patients motivated and sustained me during the more tedious aspects of this endeavor. This book's for you! Finally, thanks to my coauthor, Charlotte, for making this book a reality. You make writing fun!
—Harvey Kramer, M.D.

I want to thank all of the women who so willingly shared their stories; my friends who—sooner or later—find their experiences in my books; my dear friend Frances Chamberlain for her input; and our literary agent, Carole Abel, for her humor, patience and generous spirit.
—Charlotte Libov

I would like to thank my lovely wife, Suzanne, for her encouragement, support and tolerance of this multiyear project. I also wish to thank my children, Blake, Kendall, and Grayson, for affording me the time to work on this book. The inspiration from my many wonderful women patients motivated and sustained me during the more tedious aspects of this endeavor. This book's for you! Finally, thanks to my coauthor, Charlotte, for making this book a reality. You make writing fun!
—Harvey Kramer, M.D.

I want to thank all of the women who so willingly shared their stories; my friends who—sooner or later—find their experiences in my books; my dear friend Frances Chamberlain for her input; and our literary agent, Carole Abel, for her humor, patience and generous spirit.
—Charlotte Libov

Contents

Contents

Contents

Introduction:
How to Use This Book

As a heart attack survivor, you know that you must do everything within your power to prevent yourself from having another heart attack. The reasons are simple; as a heart attack survivor, you are at greater risk of suffering another heart attack, one that could kill you.

To prevent another heart attack, you'll need a multifaceted approach. First, you need to empower yourself, and the way to do that is to learn as much as you can about your heart, the heart attack treatments you may have undergone, and, if you've only just had your heart attack, the key steps for recuperation. You also need to know what to do in an emergency, in the event you experience another heart attack.

YOUR COMMITMENT TO CHANGE

Many women tell us they feel better now than before their heart attacks, but they've accomplished this goal after a lot of hard work. But it's not like you have a choice. You don't. You have to make these changes, because if you don't, you're more likely to

Introduction

have another heart attack. That next heart attack could kill you. It's as simple as that.

So, if you ever wanted motivation to change your lifestyle, look better, and feel better, consider this your wake-up call. But, even though your heart is going to be your Number One priority, this doesn't mean you'll be neglecting your other health concerns. Quite the opposite. If you pledge to do all you can for the health of your heart, you automatically improve your overall health and well-being.

GETTING STARTED

How do you get started on this goal-oriented approach? The great thing about goals is that they enable you to make these achievements in a "put one foot in front of the other" sort of way. As you tackle each challenge and meet each goal, your victories mount up. And each goal brings you more than the benefit of achieving it—many of these goals work synergistically, which means that their benefits add up to even more together than they do separately. So, if you control high blood pressure, diabetes, and cholesterol, you will be having an enormous impact on your risk of another heart attack, more so than achieving each of these separate goals.

YOUR TOOLS

Information: The first section of this book is all about information. We'll give you all of the information you need to know about your heart, how it works, what happened to it during your heart

Introduction

attack, the complications or damage to your heart that may have resulted, and other information you need to become empowered.

Your Doctor: We'll offer you tips on working with your doctor. Your doctor is your best ally to help you meet your goals.

Your Action Plan: Many chapters in this book—such as the ones on high blood pressure, diabetes, weight control, diet, and exercise—are filled with information on how to achieve your specific goals.

YOUR FUTURE IS BRIGHT

A heart attack can be a life-affirming wake-up call, and many women find their life afterward to be better than it was before. Not all women will find this to be true, but many of you will find that the experience is the impetus you need to make changes toward living a healthier life. This book is devoted to helping you do just that.

ONE

Women Are Different

If you're like most female heart attack survivors, you're wondering how this could have happened. Until about a decade ago, you could leaf through a medical library and conclude that virtually all of the books about heart attacks were aimed at the same audience—55-year-old males. But this was completely deceptive! Heart attacks are now—and have been for the past century—the leading cause of death in women. These heart attacks occurred not only in frail, elderly women—as you were led to expect—but in younger women in their 50s, their 40s, and even their 30s. Women just like you.

From a biological standpoint, a heart attack in a man and a woman can be very much the same. But heart attacks raise different issues for women, and it is these issues with which you must deal.

Often, when a man has a heart attack, there is an entire set of expectations that come into play. Usually a man can take time off from his job fairly easily. You may or may not be able to. But, even if you do, you may have a set of completely different responsibilities. Most women see themselves as the main caregiver in their

Chapter One

family. If you do, you may not allow yourself the recovery time you'll need.

WHY WOMEN ARE OFTEN MISDIAGNOSED

"My father died of a heart attack. My brother has had two. So, when I began experiencing pain in my arms, I decided to see the cardiologist who had treated my brother," Joyce related. "He gave me an EKG, told me it was probably stress, and told me to go to see my internist. The internist told me to go to the hospital, but once there, doctors kept dismissing my symptoms. By this time, I was sick to my stomach and they gave me Maalox. Finally, they did some tests, and when the results came in, the chief of cardiology told me I'd had a heart attack. I ended up with a lot of heart muscle damage. But they wrote on my chart that what I was experiencing during this whole time were symptoms that were not 'heart related.'"

Joyce isn't that unusual. She was a victim of a "gender myth," the belief that women do not get heart attacks. That myth is disappearing, but it still is deeply entrenched.

The Age Myth

Another reason women are so often misdiagnosed has to do with age. Yes, it's true that the majority of female heart attack victims are over the age of 65, but this bit of truth has given rise to a dangerous myth—that the hearts of younger women are immune. This is not true. Because of this myth, some women will experience heart attacks that could have been prevented if their complaints had been taken seriously.

Women Are Different

HEART ATTACK RISK FACTORS IN WOMEN

Occasionally, a woman can have a heart attack seemingly for no reason at all. But a little sleuthing will usually soon turn up reasons—known as risk factors—that account for the vast majority of heart attacks.

Simply put, a risk factor is an element proven independently to raise the risk of a heart attack.

This is the traditional list of risk factors that contribute to heart attacks in women:

- Heredity
- Age
- Smoking
- Diabetes
- High blood pressure
- Abnormal cholesterol
- Obesity
- Lack of exercise

But this list poses an obvious problem: you can't do anything about some of these risk factors. When it comes to heredity, we don't pick our parents. You can't do anything about the fact that you're growing older, or reaching menopause. These are known as "non-modifiable risk factors." But this list also includes risk factors that you can do something about. These are known as "modifiable risk factors." These include cigarette smoking, diabetes, obesity, and a sedentary lifestyle. You can also manage some of the other risk factors, including high blood pressure and abnormal cholesterol levels, through medication and lifestyle change.

Not long ago, these risk factors were believed to account for about 50 percent of all heart attacks. But now we know that four of these risk factors account for a whopping 80 percent of heart attacks. These "big four" are:

- Smoking
- Abnormal cholesterol
- Diabetes
- High blood pressure

Also, the younger you were when you had your heart attack, the more likely it was caused by one or more of these four risk factors. This doesn't mean that heart attacks never happen to women who do not have these heart disease risk factors. But for women who do not have these risk factors, heart attacks occur much more rarely than previously thought. This also doesn't mean the other risk factors enumerated in that longer list aren't important—they are. In fact, some of them play into the major ones. For instance, obesity and a lack of activity are major contributors to that "super" risk factor—diabetes.

RISK FACTORS YOU CAN CHANGE

What is also very important about the "big four" risk factors is that they are risk factors you can control.

Smoking

Smoking is the most dangerous thing you can do to your heart. Smoking is considered responsible for half of the heart attacks in women under the age of 55, and women who smoke are up to 3 times more likely to suffer a heart attack than those who don't smoke. For women who started smoking before the age of 15, the risk is even greater. Not surprisingly, the risk is highest for the heaviest of smokers, but light smokers aren't off the hook either.

Smoking damages your heart in two ways. First, toxic chemicals that are contained in cigarette smoke damage the walls of your coronary arteries, setting the stage for coronary artery disease. Second, tobacco smoke has blood-clotting properties, and blood clots are the ultimate cause of heart attacks.

These dangers exist even if you choose "low-tar" and "low-nicotine" cigarettes. In fact, since low-nicotine cigarettes may not satisfy a smoker's cravings, she may smoke more of them.

Abnormal Cholesterol

Cholesterol is an essential substance found in our bodies. But having the wrong amounts of the components can raise your heart attack risk. Your doctor generally evaluates four types of cholesterol: total cholesterol, good cholesterol (HDL or high-density lipoprotein), bad cholesterol (LDL or low-density lipoprotein), and triglyceride (a storage form of fat in the body). The total cholesterol, when you are fasting, is the sum of these other three components (HDL + LDL + TG/5). Analyzing all of these components gives the most complete description of your cholesterol pattern.

Diabetes

Diabetes is an extremely powerful risk factor for heart attacks in women. In fact, it's estimated that the death rate from heart attacks among women with diabetes is two to four times higher than for women without diabetes. Women with diabetes are about 400 percent more likely to suffer a heart attack. Furthermore, women who develop diabetes before menopause have the same risk of suffering a heart attack that men in this age group do. This means that diabetes erases what has been called the "gender protection period" for women. Diabetes also raises the probability of developing other risk factors, such as high blood pressure and abnormal lipids, which affect the blood cholesterol balance. Diabetes also poses an additional danger to women who have had heart attacks. Diabetes causes changes in the nerve cells, which can result in your body's misinterpreting pain signals, such as chest pain. You're at increased risk of experiencing a heart attack that you are not even aware of because you may not feel any pain.

High Blood Pressure

About 25 million women in America have high blood pressure. High blood pressure raises the risk of a heart attack because it increases the force of your blood against your delicate blood vessels, which can damage them. Although high blood pressure raises your risk for another heart attack, it raises your risk of stroke even more. Since no one wants a stroke either, treating high blood pressure is an important part of your recovery plan.

The Metabolic Syndrome

Another way of looking at dangerous risk factors is to consider the "metabolic syndrome," a set of conditions that tend to cluster together, dramatically increasing heart attack risk.

Women with this syndrome have at least three of the following conditions:

- Obesity (a waist measurement of more than 35 inches).
- Abnormal blood cholesterol (triglyceride levels in the blood of 150 or greater and HDL, or "good" cholesterol, of less than 50).
- High blood pressure (a blood pressure reading of 130/85 or greater).
- Impaired fasting glucose (a fasting blood sugar level of 100 or more).

A healthy diet, exercise, and medication can help improve these conditions and reduce your risk. Even losing just a relatively small amount of weight can bring about a significant improvement.

Potential Heart Disease Risk Factors

It's now known that the currently identified risk factors account for most—but not all—heart attacks. Also, even if you have risk factors, it isn't completely known what triggers the heart attack process itself. Elevated levels of certain substances in the blood are suspect. These include fibrinogen (a type of protein), homocystine (an amino acid), and iron. Lesser-known dietary factors, such as drinking strong, unfiltered coffee, have been linked. So has sleeping more than eight hours a day—or sleeping less. Some of these risk factors may emerge more strongly in the future, and others will be disproved.

One of these lesser-known risk factors currently gaining attention is C-reactive protein (CRP), which is a protein produced by the liver in response to inflammation that may be linked to heart disease, especially in women. Recently, it has become practical to check the blood's CRP levels, thanks to a new, more sensitive test. This new test can be requested whenever blood is

Chapter One

drawn for other tests. The cost can vary greatly, from $17 to $250 per test, depending on insurance coverage and the volume of tests performed at a particular lab.

But a number of questions exist. It isn't known, for instance, if CRP is a marker for heart disease (meaning that it's basically an innocent bystander), or whether it is a cause of the disease. It also isn't known whether taking steps to lower CRP has any sort of beneficial result. Still, if you are searching for a cause for your heart attack and your doctor is at a loss to explain it, you might want to consider the blood test.

Just as there is much that is known about major risk factors, there are still some aspects of heart disease risk factors that remain a mystery. In the meantime, don't let this deter you from fighting the known risk factors that result in the vast majority of heart attacks. Identifying your risk factors and working to change them can help you prevent having another heart attack.

HORMONES AND YOUR HEART

As a woman, your hormones are part of the equation when you're seeking to protect your heart. Your age plays a role, of course. How your hormones affect your body—and also what you do regarding hormonal replacement—depends on your stage of life. Here's the information you need to help you make these decisions.

Contraception

If you're past menopause—which means you haven't gotten your period for a full year—birth control is not a concern for you. But if you are still able to conceive, it is. Although contraceptives—whether taken orally or in a form such as the birth control patch—are generally safe for most women, this is not true for heart attack survivors.

Birth control pills are generally made up of two hormones: progestin (a synthetic form of the hormone progesterone) and estrogen. When oral contraceptives were first marketed in the 1970s, they raised the risk of blood clots in apparently healthy women, resulting in heart attacks, strokes, and pulmonary embolis (blood clots that lodge in the arteries of the lungs). Over the years, new formulations were developed, reducing this risk. However, the added risk for heart attack survivors still remains, whether the hormones are taken orally, injected, implanted under the skin, or administered by way of a patch. So, if birth control is of concern to you, you should consider using another means, such as condoms or a "barrier" method of birth control (for example, a diaphragm, a cervical cap, or a contraceptive sponge).

How Menopause Increases Heart Attack Risk

As both men and women grow older, their heart attack risk increases. For women, this increased risk coincides with menopause.

Menopause, the time when your reproductive cycle comes to an end, usually occurs between 41 to 55 years of age, with an average age of 51. If you've had your ovaries removed surgically, or received chemotherapy and/or radiation, you may experience "premature menopause," which means that your reproductive cycle has ended earlier than it would have normally.

A woman's heart attack risk increases as she ages, and it coincides with the years of menopause. It is not known exactly what raises this heart attack risk, but it's been assumed for some time to be connected with the decline in estrogen (the so-called female sex hormone), which occurs at this time. Once, estrogen was thought to primarily affect a woman's reproductive system, but it is now becoming clear that estrogen may affect almost every other organ of the body as well, including the brain, breasts, heart, urinary tract, and bones.

The Changing View of Replacement Hormones

Hormone replacement therapy was developed in an attempt to prevent the negative effects that menopause—and the decline of estrogen—appeared to bring with it. These effects include such symptoms as hot flashes and vaginal dryness. Such symptoms are now more accurately described as "perimenopausal," which means that these symptoms generally occur in the years when a woman's reproductive cycle is "winding down" and heading toward menopause.

Two approaches to hormone replacement are:

- *Estrogen replacement therapy (ERT):* This refers to the practice of giving pure (known as "unopposed") estrogen.
- *Hormone replacement therapy (HRT):* This is a combination of estrogen and progestin and is the more widely used form of replacement therapy. There are several such combination preparations on the market.

The idea of supplementing hormones in aging women isn't new; it goes back to the 1920s. Using hormone therapy as a way to stay young was popularized in the 1970s, but it was eventually found that giving pure estrogen to women increased their risk of uterine cancer, which is also known as endometrial cancer. Researchers found that combining estrogen with progestin, a synthetic form of progesterone, reduced this risk. Progesterone is the other reproductive hormone, which is produced along with estrogen. The estrogen and progestin combination, known as HRT, became the standard type of replacement therapy used for women who had not had a hysterectomy and therefore retained their uterus.

The Food and Drug Administration has approved HRT for menopausal symptoms, such as hot flashes, and for the prevention of osteoporosis, and a large-scale study, the Women's Health Initiative (WHI), was begun to determine if it prevented heart disease (which it seemed to). But that study was halted in 2002, when it was found that instead of preventing heart attacks, HRT actually increased risk. Two years later, it was found that women who were taking estrogen, not the combination, also did not benefit. So, when it comes to preventing heart disease, hormone replacement has not proven to be the answer.

Finding Relief from Menopause Symptoms

If you are suffering from menopausal symptoms, such as hot flashes, talk to your doctor about taking the lowest possible dosage of hormones for the shortest period of time for the relief of your symptoms. The problem, though, is that there is no proof that shows how low a dose or how short a time is safe. As results from the WHI continue to come in, it's becoming clear that the risk of heart attacks began to rise during the first year that the women were taking the drug, and that risk also occurred in the younger women. But it wasn't necessarily the heart attack risk that halted the study. The study also found that for the women who developed breast cancer, theirs was a dangerous, invasive type of disease, putting to bed the myth that such "hormone-caused cancers" were less harmful.

Chapter One

So, you need to weigh the pros and cons of HRT for yourself. If your menopausal symptoms are unrelenting, perhaps it's worth the risk. But bear in mind that you'll also be increasing your heart attack risk, so if you can manage it, you'd probably be best off steering clear of HRT.

Hormone Alternatives

Many women suffering from the symptoms of menopause turn to "natural" hormones in the mistaken belief that if it's natural, it must be safe. Unfortunately, that isn't necessarily the case. Also, these medications are not regulated, nor are they subject to the kind of vigorous testing that ERT and HRT underwent. Generally, no matter where hormones come from—be they animal hormones, like the type studied in the WHI, or plant-based hormones—if they act like hormones, they most likely carry the same risks as hormones.

There is one non-hormonal remedy that some women report may help hot flashes, and that is aerobic exercise. Since that's also good for your heart, it's one approach that's easy to enthusiastically recommend.

TWO

How the Heart Works

To prevent another heart attack, it's important to understand the structure of your heart and how it functions. This way, you can better understand what damage may have occurred during your heart attack, as well as how medication and surgical procedures can help to strengthen your heart.

A BIG JOB FOR A SMALL ORGAN

Your heart is about the shape and size of your closed fist. The job of your heart is to keep blood pumping throughout your body. This is blood that carries oxygen and nutrients to all your organs, which need it to survive.

This is no easy task, because your body contains about 60,000 miles of blood vessels, and your heart must keep this blood pumping all the time, without a rest, for your entire life. To accomplish this, your heart needs to "beat" (or expand and contract). Your heart does this about 100,000 times each day, pumping about 2,000 gallons of blood, bringing the needed blood to your brain, kidneys, lungs, and all your other organs.

Chapter Two

YOUR HEART:
ITS STRUCTURE AND FUNCTIONS

Your heart is a four-chambered, hollow organ composed of cardiac muscle, a tough type of muscle found only in the heart. The heart is divided into two sides, right and left, by a muscular wall known as the *septum*. The two sides are further divided into two top chambers, the *atria*, and two bottom chambers, *the ventricles*. The two sides work in concert as the blood travels along, receiving oxygen from the lungs, and then the oxygenated blood is pumped back to the rest of the body.

It is extremely important that the blood travels correctly, in forward fashion. Four valves make sure this happens. They function very much as "safety valves," preventing the blood from leaking backward and going in the wrong direction. These four valves are the *tricuspid valve*, the *pulmonic valve*, the *mitral valve*, and the *aortic valve*. As it makes its way to the heart and lungs, the blood travels through specific vessels. First, the unoxygenated blood enters your heart on the right side, through two major blood vessels: *the superior vena cava* and the *inferior vena cava*. The blood then flows through the right heart chambers, to the pulmonary artery, which delivers the blood to the lungs, where it is infused with oxygen. Then, it flows to the left side of the heart, from the lungs via the *pulmonary veins*, where it is then pumped out of the heart to the rest of the body.

Since the heart is also a living organ, it must receive oxygen from the blood as well. Providing oxygenated blood to the heart is the vital job of your coronary arteries. They are located on the outside of the heart muscle, and they are very thin, like strands of spaghetti. Therefore, any narrowing of them can impede this blood supply, causing serious trouble.

How the Heart Works

HOW HEART ATTACKS HAPPEN
Coronary Artery Disease

Most commonly, a heart attack occurs because of a blood clot, which blocks the vital flow of blood to the heart and deprives it of its needed oxygen supply. Usually, this blood clot is the end result of coronary artery disease, known also as coronary heart disease or, more technically, as atherosclerosis. This disease process causes the heart's coronary arteries to become narrowed with plaque, a substance made from cholesterol and other fatty materials. If a bit of this plaque breaks, ruptures, or erodes, a blood clot forms at this site and blocks the artery, resulting in a heart attack.

Still, the mere presence of plaque in the arteries doesn't necessarily result in a heart attack. Plaque can become hardened (calcified) and narrow the artery, but it can remain stable, with no clot occurring. This narrowing deprives the heart of some of its oxygen, but not all of it. So, when you are active and your heart needs more oxygen, symptoms of this lack of oxygen can occur, like chest pain or shortness of breath. This condition is known as "stable angina," angina being the medical term for chest pain that comes from a heart-related cause. If this condition grows worse, and a clot seems likely to form, or a small clot has already formed, this condition is known as "unstable angina." This condition requires prompt treatment because it can be the harbinger of a heart attack.

Coronary Spasms

A heart attack can also be caused by a coronary spasm. This means that a coronary artery has become temporarily dangerously constricted. This condition is a less common cause of heart attacks than atherosclerotic coronary artery disease, but it does occur more frequently in women, and in men and women who smoke. Coronary spasm with dissection, or tearing of the artery, is also often the culprit in the rare cases of pregnant women who suffer heart attacks.

Women who have generally plaque-free arteries can suffer a heart attack due to a coronary spasm. However, on occasion, a woman with coronary artery disease can suffer a heart attack caused by a coronary spasm in the region of an artery partially narrowed by plaque.

Other Heart Attack Causes

A very tiny percentage of heart attacks—around 5 percent—occur from other causes, such as severe anemia, an aortic dissection (a tear in the aorta), or an extremely serious acute illness. But these heart attack causes occur exceedingly uncommonly.

UNCOMPLICATED VS. COMPLICATED HEART ATTACKS

During a heart attack, your heart muscle is deprived of blood for a certain amount of time, causing some heart damage. If the heart attack has no other associated problems with it, this is known as an "uncomplicated" heart attack. Fortunately, uncomplicated heart attacks are now the most common type, thanks to treatments that quickly restore blood flow to the heart. If, however, enough heart damage occurs to cause additional problems, this is known as a "complicated" heart attack.

The two main complications that can occur after a heart attack are *arrhythmias* and *congestive heart failure*. An arrhythmia is an irregular heartbeat. Different types of arrhythmias can occur during and after a heart attack. Congestive heart failure occurs when the heart is not able to circulate adequate amounts of blood. This can result in an accumulation of fluids in any part of the body, but most commonly in the lungs, legs, and feet.

Rare Heart Attack Complications

A number of other serious complications can occur during or after a heart attack, but fortunately, they are rare. Some can be life threatening and require emergency treatment. Here is a rundown, in alphabetical order:

Cerebral Embolism

Rarely, after a heart attack, a blood clot can form on the inside of the heart muscle. If the heart's pumping mechanism is impaired, this can result in the formation of a clot, which can adhere to the wall of the heart. Sometimes, this can occur even if the overall pumping action is normal. If a bit of this clot comes loose and travels to the brain, the result is a cerebral embolism, or stroke. The symptoms of a stroke include temporary or permanent impairment or weakness on one side of the body, problems with balance and coordination, difficulty with speech or memory, vision problems, dizziness or numbness, trouble thinking, and sudden fatigue. Strokes are treated with medication to dissolve the clot, blood thinners, or, less commonly, with surgery. Rehabilitation may also be part of the treatment.

Mitral Regurgitation

The mitral valve, one of your heart's four valves, ensures that your blood flows through the heart properly, from the upper to the lower chamber. It is attached to the heart by two papillary muscles, which anchor it to the heart wall. If these muscles are damaged during the heart attack, this may result in mitral regurgitation, which is also known as mitral insufficiency. This is, basically, a leaky valve, which causes some of the blood to flow backward, in the wrong direction. This causes the heart to overwork. Symptoms can include shortness of breath, fatigue, and weakness. This condition can also lead to other complications, most notably congestive heart failure. When this leakage occurs suddenly, from damage during a heart attack, the symptoms can be severe. If needed, surgery can be performed to repair or replace the damaged mitral valve.

Pericarditis or Dressler's Syndrome

This less serious complication is an inflammation of the pericardium, which is the translucent sac that surrounds the heart and the roots of the coronary arteries. The cause is not known but is thought to be possibly due to the body's autoimmune response. The symptom is chest pain that is particularly sharp and knife-like, especially upon taking a deep breath. Sitting up and leaning forward may help decrease the pain. It usually occurs four or five days after a heart attack, but it can occur up to six weeks afterward. This is usually not a life-threatening complication, but it causes great distress, because it can be mistakenly assumed that the chest pain heralds another heart attack. This condition is treated with medication.

Pulmonary Embolism

A pulmonary embolism, or clot in the lung, can occur if a blood clot forms either in the right side of the heart or, more commonly, in the pelvis or legs and travels through the right side of the heart to the lungs. Symptoms may include a cough, shortness of breath, chest pain, rapid breathing, and a rapid heart rate. In severe cases, shock and heart failure can occur. In cases of very large pulmonary clots, emergency medication to dissolve the clot is administered, although sometimes surgery is necessary.

Ventricular Aneurysm

This complication can occur after a heart attack in which a large area of heart muscle is damaged. The damaged muscle is replaced by thin scar tissue, which pushes out part of the heart wall as the heart is beating. This enlarges the ventricle, which is the heart's main pumping chamber. This may result in irregular heartbeat rhythms, recurrent chest pain, and congestive heart failure. This aneurysm causes a situation in which a blood clot can form and travel to the brain, causing a stroke. It is very rare that this part of the heart muscle would actually tear, or rupture. This complication may not cause any symptoms, but it may be detected during a follow-up exam. Unless it is severe, the condition is usually treated with cardiac drugs to correct the irregular heart rhythms and prevent blood clots from forming. Severe cases may require surgery to remove the dead heart muscle and sew the remaining healthy parts together. This is usually performed in conjunction with a coronary bypass operation.

Ventricular Septal Rupture and Ventricular Free Wall Rupture

These are two serious, rare complications that involve the left side of the heart, which is the main pumping chamber. They must be surgically corrected.

Ventricular septal rupture typically occurs within two weeks following a heart attack. A rupture, or actual hole, occurs in the

Chapter Two

heart muscle, at the margin of the heart attack, where the damaged heart muscle meets the normal heart muscle. The blood stays within the chambers of the heart, overloading them with too much blood and pressure, resulting in a sharp drop in blood pressure and heart failure. A new, loud heart murmur (abnormal heart sound) is also heard.

A ventricular free wall rupture usually occurs in the front or side of the left ventricle (the main pumping chamber of the heart) and is a slit-like tear in the heart muscle at the junction of muscle damaged by the heart attack and normal muscle. This allows blood to leak out of the heart into the pericardial sac, which is the membrane surrounding the heart. If the leakage is very small, no symptoms may occur. However, if the leakage is large, and especially if it has occurred rapidly, the blood pools in the pericardium and rapidly builds up high blood pressure around the heart. This results in a drop in blood pressure and may quickly result in total collapse (cardiogenic shock).

THREE

How to Know It's a Heart Attack

The telltale chest pain of a heart attack comes on over the space of a minute or two, builds in intensity, lasts for at least 20 minutes, and is not relieved by rest or by changing position. The pain itself can range from mild to severe, or it may manifest itself more as a feeling of pressure or heaviness. The pain also can radiate into your jaw, your back, or down your left arm. Other symptoms can include nausea, sweating, shortness of breath, or a sense of impending doom.

Male heart attack survivors describe symptoms that have a certain similarity: a feeling of crushing chest pain and pressure, for instance. Women sometimes recount similar symptoms, but other times, their accounts can differ widely. The point is that women do not always experience the classic heart attack symptoms that men often describe.

For Alison, for instance, the commonly cited symptom of chest pain played a role in her symptoms, which she recalls in this way:

"That night, I awoke at 3 a.m. The pain woke me up. It was unbelievable, going from my throat to my diaphragm. I drank an entire bottle of Mylanta and I was able to go back to sleep. But, when I got up at 6 a.m., I was actually whimpering. I started throwing up a little later, which made me think it was a gastrointestinal problem. By the time I got to our local hospital and I was checked in, it felt that someone had wrapped a band around my ribs. There was constant pressure. It hurt so much that if you told me you were going to put a hot knife to my chest and get rid of what was causing the pain, I would have said, 'Go ahead.'"

But Karen's experience was much different:

"I can't remember honestly if I felt anything before I went to bed, but I woke up at about 3 a.m. It felt like my throat and esophagus were really raw and there was tightness under my collarbone. I decided I felt weird enough that I would go to the emergency room and they would examine me and send me home. I took a shower and, looking in the mirror, realized my color wasn't right; I was definitely paler than usual. So I went into the emergency room and, as I was answering questions, I started getting nauseous."

HEART ATTACK SYMPTOMS: MEN VS. WOMEN

Here's a recap of the common symptoms of heart attack:

- Chest pain
- Pain that may radiate into the jaw, back, or down the left arm
- Shortness of breath
- Nausea, sweating
- A feeling of impending doom

Keep in mind that, for the good part of a century, the symptoms most often experienced by men became associated with all heart attacks. This is because virtually all the medical research used in compiling them was done on men. And the main symptom seemed to be pain or pressure that occurred in the region of the chest. It's only within the past few years that any significant research on heart attacks in women has been done, and those results are just now coming in.

So, although women may experience chest pain and other heart attack symptoms that have been described by men for ages, it's becoming clear that women are more likely to experience subtle symptoms, such as the following:

- Indigestion
- Chest discomfort
- Unusual tiredness or shortness of breath

SYMPTOMS THAT MIMIC HEART ATTACKS

Virtually all women experience chest pain at some point in their lives, and for many of them, the cause has nothing to do with their hearts. As a heart attack survivor, having pain in your chest may make you understandably concerned. You do need to get it checked out. On the other hand, women, even more so than men, are prone to chest pain due to a variety of non-heart-related sources. Here, in alphabetical order, is a rundown on the conditions that can cause chest pain resembling the type that occurs during a heart attack:

Esophageal Dysfunction

Also known as esophageal reflux, this condition occurs when food that should be moving through your esophagus to the stomach does not continue to pass through normally, causing some of the acidic contents to splash back. This irritates the esophagus and causes a sensation most of us know as "heartburn," but it can also sometimes feel like chest pain. Often, but not always, esophageal reflux is seen in women who are overweight. Smoking, anxiety, alcohol, caffeine, and heavy meals can aggravate this condition as well. Treatment usually includes watching your diet, losing weight, and taking medication.

Gas

The common problem of intestinal gas can mimic heart-related chest pain. Excessive gas can be caused by irritable bowel syndrome (also called spastic colon), which is accompanied by alternating periods of diarrhea and constipation. Another source of excessive gas is lactose intolerance, in which your body is unable to digest the lactose, or milk sugar, found in dairy products. This condition also causes cramps, bloating, and diarrhea. Eating a dairy-free diet is the best way to ease symptoms from lactose intolerance.

Muscular Pain

Women who are large-breasted can experience chest pain. You can also get chest pain from problems arising from the muscular and skeletal structure of the chest. Sometimes, for instance, when your ribs rub against each other in the course of normal movement, their joints can become inflamed, which causes a painful condition known as "costochondritis." (This condition can also be caused by a virus that can follow a flu-like illness.) There are medications available to treat this problem.

Osteoarthritis of the Neck

Osteoarthritis is the most common form of arthritis. Usually associated with the elderly, it can occur in younger women as well. Although it sounds odd, this is one of the most common causes of chest pain in women. Osteoarthritis of the neck causes bony spurs, which can be seen on a neck x-ray. The condition can cause "referred pain," which is felt in the chest. Treatments include anti-inflammatory drugs, heat, neck traction, or other types of physical therapy.

Shingles

Known medically as "herpes zoster," shingles causes not only the painful rash that is associated with it, but also chest pain. You can only get shingles if you had chickenpox in the past; after you have chickenpox, the virus lies dormant in the nerves. The disease generally manifests itself when you get older (especially when you are over 50), or if you have a weakened immune system. Shingles is a very painful disease, but there are medications that can offer relief.

BETTER SAFE THAN SORRY

It is important to remember that all of these conditions can manifest symptoms similar to chest pain. If you know you have one of these problems or your symptoms disappear after the appropriate treatment (taking antacids after a heavy meal, for instance), that's great. But, if you suspect your symptoms may be heart-related, have your doctor check them out. Better to be safe than sorry.

GETTING TO THE HOSPITAL

As a heart attack survivor, you're at higher risk for another one. So you should have an emergency plan in place in case you experience symptoms that lead you to believe you might be having another heart attack. This will give you peace of mind. Here are the items for your emergency plan:

- Call 911. Never attempt to drive yourself to the hospital. The ride from home to a hospital in an ambulance will be faster than driving yourself and, if necessary, medical care can be administered immediately on the way.
- Tell the 911 dispatcher that you are a heart attack survivor, and you suspect that you are having another heart attack.
- Give your exact street location. Make certain your house is posted with a clearly visible number, and specify the floor, room, or apartment number.
- Turn on the outside lights if it's night, and make sure the door is unlocked.
- Call your cardiologist immediately. Your cardiologist's phone number should be kept by every telephone in the house. Discuss with your cardiologist beforehand whether he or she may be best contacted at the office or at the clinic or hospital.
- If you arrive at the hospital's emergency room on your own, clearly state that you may be suffering a heart attack, and let them know that you've had one before. This is especially important for women, since heart disease is sometimes overlooked in women. If it turns out you are not having a heart attack, that's all the better. But go to the hospital—don't attempt to diagnose the problem yourself.

FOUR

What Happens in the Hospital

EMERGENCY CARE

The care you receive begins immediately, as emergency workers stabilize your condition at home and in the ambulance. At the hospital, many heart attack sufferers are admitted through the emergency room and then are transferred to the Coronary Care Unit (CCU). The CCU is an area in which heart attack sufferers can be further evaluated and closely monitored. There, a specially trained nurse who works with doctors and other members of the medical team provides individualized care.

The length of stay in the CCU varies, depending on the severity of your heart attack, what treatment you received (for example, angioplasty), whether or not you experienced complications, and if so, how serious they are. If your heart attack occurred without complications, you probably spent about two to three days in the CCU before being transferred to a step-down unit. A step-down unit offers less intensive care than the CCU but still generally provides continuous monitoring to screen for abnormal heart rhythms or other complications. Whether you are discharged from

Chapter Four

the step-down unit or after being transferred to a regular floor depends on your clinical course as well as on the hospital's policy.

Monitoring your heart after a heart attack is very necessary. During a heart attack and immediately afterward, your blood pressure can shoot too high or fall too low; your heart's internal electrical system, which regulates your heartbeat, can go haywire, sending your heart racing irregularly or slowing it down too much. Cardiac units have equipment and staff to quickly identify and counteract such occurrences and stabilize your condition.

DIAGNOSING THE HEART ATTACK

If there is any doubt whether you had a heart attack, tests will be done to confirm it. These include blood tests to check the level of cardiac enzymes, which are used to confirm the diagnosis. Once the diagnosis of a heart attack is confirmed, treatment begins almost instantaneously. Even before it is definitively confirmed, treatment may start if there is a high degree of suspicion that a heart attack is occurring.

Testing Your Heart

When you were brought to the hospital, diagnostic tests were performed to definitively determine if you were having a heart attack and, if so, how to minimize the damage and ensure you survive it. But tests were also done to determine what kind of heart attack you were having, how much damage occurred, and how this would affect your future health. Years ago, it was standard practice to perform a number of tests spread out over a period of time to get this information. Nowadays, these tests are compressed into a much shorter period of time, usually within the first few days of hospitalization. Because heart attacks are now treated more aggressively, such information is needed sooner.

The type of information these tests furnish is important for you to know, because cardiac testing will be an important part of your life from now on. How often and which tests you need will depend on your individual condition. If you recover normally, you may only need to return for follow-up testing infrequently. But if you experience recurrent symptoms, or if you or your doctor suspects you may be developing complications (problems that occur due to heart damage), you may require additional tests.

The initial tests done at the time of emergency treatment may be repeated during your hospitalization to provide your doctors with more information, such as how much of your heart muscle was damaged, whether complications are likely to occur, and how well you responded to treatment. These same tests may be repeated again after you are discharged and during your follow-up doctor visits.

The following tests are done to diagnose or confirm whether or not you've had a heart attack, to assess any damage to your heart, or to ascertain which types of treatments are recommended.

Electrocardiogram

An electrocardiogram (EKG or ECG) measures the electrical signals that reflect the structure and function of both the electrical and muscular systems of your heart. The results are displayed graphically, on a printout. By reading it, your doctor can tell the size of the chambers of your heart, whether your heart rhythms are normal, whether the electrical circuits of your heart are working properly, and whether your heart may have suffered any muscle damage from a previous heart attack. But although the EKG can provide valuable information, it is not uncommon for these test results to appear normal, or nearly so, especially during the early stages of a heart attack. This is why the next test, a cardiac protein blood test, is also needed to confirm whether or not you had a heart attack.

Cardiac Protein Blood Tests

Cardiac protein blood tests detect the telltale presence of certain types of substances in the blood that are the result of a heart attack. During a heart attack, the heart muscle releases a specific protein, known as troponin, and a cardiac enzyme, known as creatine phosphokinase (CPK or CK). There are tests done to measure either substance, but the troponin test is believed to be more specific than CPK because troponin is found only in the heart muscle, while CPK enzymes can be found in other tissues as well. The troponin is also more sensitive in detecting a smaller amount of heart muscle damage than the CPK. Tests using troponin are so sensitive that they can pick up heart attacks that previously went undiagnosed, and in fact, these tests are responsible for changing the way a heart attack is defined. Ten years ago, many people who suffered chest pain were told that they had not experienced a heart attack, because no changes in the EKG or CPK would have been noted. Nowadays, they would be classified as having a heart attack, thanks to this ultrasensitive test.

Troponin and cardiac enzyme tests are also sometimes repeated after an angioplasty or coronary artery bypass surgery, to determine if any damage occurred to the heart muscle as a result of these procedures. These tests can also be used to identify who is at higher risk for future heart attacks and heart problems.

What Happens in the Hospital

Echocardiogram

Like an EKG, an echocardiogram is also a commonly performed cardiac diagnostic test that is routinely done following a heart attack to determine the extent of damage done. For this test, a technician places EKG leads on your chest and then moves a probe around the outside of your chest wall to visualize the heart with sound waves. The probe sends high-pitched sound waves, which produce a moving image of the structures of your heart and the manner in which your blood flows through it.

An echocardiogram also produces a measurement known as an "ejection fraction," which shows how strong your heart is pumping. The test shows how well your heart chambers fill with blood, and the efficiency with which it is pumped to the rest of the body. An ejection fraction of at least 50 percent is considered efficient. A score of less than 40 percent may indicate that treatment is needed to prevent your heart muscle from deteriorating further. An echocardiogram can also show whether or not the heart is enlarged (another possible complication following a heart attack), whether there is any evidence of previous heart attacks, and how well your heart valves function. This test can also help identify areas of the heart that are not receiving enough blood, the hallmark of a heart attack and heart muscle damage.

A "transesophageal echocardiogram" is a variation of an echocardiogram that is used when a traditional "transthoracic" echocardiogram cannot provide clear enough images. This happens when a woman is particularly large-breasted or very overweight, or when a woman has particularly severe lung disease, for example. For this test, you swallow a small version of the probe used in a traditional echocardiogram. The probe then rests inside

Chapter Four

the esophagus, behind the heart, where it provides a clear view of your heart from directly behind it.

Exercise Stress Test

Before being discharged, you will most likely undergo some type of exercise stress test to determine whether the flow of blood to your heart is unobstructed and how likely it is that you may suffer another heart attack in the near future. A good result shows you are not in danger of having another heart attack, and you can safely go home. You will probably be rescheduled in few weeks for another stress test, where you'll exercise more strenuously. This test is done to make sure that your heart is receiving enough blood, enabling you to resume your normal activities. This test will be repeated periodically, even after you've recovered.

An exercise stress test combines an EKG with physical activity, such as walking on a treadmill or riding a stationary bike. Leads are attached to your chest, as in a regular EKG, to monitor changes in your heartbeat. You begin exercising at a slow pace that gradually speeds up.

Although this type of simple test is a major diagnostic tool for men, it is less accurate when used on women, although the reason for this is not clearly understood. So you'll undergo one of these two variations: an exercise test with an imaging agent, or an exercise echocardiogram, which combines an exercise test with an echocardiogram.

These types of exercise tests provide your doctor with important information, including whether your heart is receiving adequate blood flow and how well your heart muscle is pumping. Sometimes, you may not have any chest pain when lying in bed, but it comes on during exercise. These tests can show whether the pain is being caused by a coronary artery that has remained dangerously narrowed. Some people may have no further pain at all but may, nevertheless, have inadequate blood flow to the heart, as demonstrated by the stress test. This "silent ischemia" can be dangerous, even without symptoms of pain.

Your doctor can also use the information to determine which medications you should be taking, and also to write you an exercise "prescription," or plan, so that you can perform the right physical exercises to further improve your heart's function and efficiency, and improve your overall level of fitness and well-being.

Both of these types of exercise stress tests furnish the same type of information, so which one is used depends on the type that is preferred where you undergo it. The exercise stress test with nuclear imaging has been around longer than the exercise echocardiogram, so it is more commonly performed.

This is also the test you'll probably undergo if you are experiencing symptoms similar to those that preceded your heart attack, so your doctor can ascertain if your coronary arteries have remained clear or are becoming renarrowed.

Exercise Stress Test with Imaging

An exercise stress test with imaging is similar to a regular exercise stress test, but an imaging agent is given to you, intravenously, to provide images of your heart. This enables your doctor to better evaluate the blood flow through your coronary arteries.

Exercise Echocardiogram

For this test, a baseline echocardiogram is performed. Once the baseline results are established, you exercise on a treadmill or on a stationary bicycle, just as you would during an exercise stress test.

After this portion of the test, a repeat echocardiogram is performed, and the results of the two tests are compared to determine whether your heart is receiving an adequate blood flow.

Pharmacological Stress Test

If you have a physical problem, such as severe arthritis, which prevents you from exercising, you may undergo a "pharmacological stress test." This test provides the necessary information about your heart without your doing much or any exercise at all. In this case, a drug, such as dipyridamole or adenosine, is administered intravenously. These medications affect the coronary arteries. Images of your heart are then taken. If the vessels are normal, the drug will cause them to widen, which they won't be able to do if they've been narrowed by coronary artery disease.

Coronary Angiogram

Also known as cardiac catheterization, a coronary angiogram can be done on an emergency basis, while you are experiencing your heart attack, to determine whether angioplasty or coronary bypass surgery is needed. This test is always done before any type of surgical cardiac procedure, such as angioplasty or coronary bypass surgery, because the results furnish your doctor with the extent and location of the narrowing and blockages in the coronary arteries that are impeding the flow of blood to your heart.

Because it's now more commonly available than in the past, heart attack patients may undergo angioplasty immediately, so it is possible you have already undergone an angiogram during the initial treatment for your heart attack. However, if you were administered a clot-busting drug, instead of undergoing an angioplasty, or if you did not undergo either treatment, you may be sent for an angiogram, especially if you are still experiencing symptoms, if your symptoms recur, or if other diagnostic tests indicate some potentially dangerous artery-narrowing plaque remaining in your coronary arteries.

This procedure is done in the hospital, so if you've already been discharged, you'll return and undergo it as an outpatient. Most small hospitals are not equipped to perform this test; if this is the case, you'll be referred to a larger institution.

An angiogram is performed while you are awake but sedated. The catheter is usually inserted by way of the femoral artery, a large accessible artery in the groin. An artery in the arm is sometimes used: either the artery in front of your elbow (the brachial artery) or the artery in the wrist (the radial artery). Once the catheter is in place, the physician guides it to the vicinity of the site where the coronary arteries branch off the aorta to the heart. Then dye is injected and traces the route of the blood flow, pinpointing any obstructions.

After the procedure, you will most likely spend the next several hours resting. If your femoral artery was used, heavy pressure, which can be quite uncomfortable, may be applied for about twenty minutes to close the artery. A relatively new device, which actually promotes the formation of a blood clot at the site of the catheter insertion, can be used to "plug" it, shortening the recovery period. If your arm was used for the catheter, you may be able to get up sooner and be discharged earlier.

Intravascular Ultrasound

In the vast majority of cases, a coronary angiogram, which precisely pinpoints the location of arterial narrowing or blockages, provides sufficient information. Sometimes, though, more information is needed about such blockages. In this case, a test known as an intravascular ultrasound may be performed.

For this test, a miniature sound probe, similar to (but tinier than) that used for an echocardiogram, is attached to the end of a catheter and threaded into the coronary arteries during the angiogram to see inside the vessel. This test is also sometimes used after an angioplasty to make certain that, if a stent was deployed during the procedure, it is properly positioned. This is also useful for women who experience severe chest pain and whose coronary arteries appear normal on an angiogram but who, in fact, are found to have narrowed arteries when examined by this newer technology.

DIAGNOSING COMPLICATIONS

Damage to your heart caused by a heart attack can cause complications. Two of the most common problems are arrhythmias, or heart rhythm disturbances, and congestive heart failure, which is a condition created when the heart is not able to circulate adequate amounts of blood throughout the body. These are the tests used to diagnose these conditions:

Ambulatory Electrocardiographic Monitoring

Damage from a heart attack can result in your developing an arrhythmia, or irregular heartbeat. These can occur when you are not in the doctor's office, so a number of different devices have been developed that record your heartbeat as you go about your daily activities.

Holtor monitor: This is the most well known. You wear this device, which is a bit larger than a deck of cards, for 24–48 hours, to produce an EKG recording of every heartbeat. You may also be told to keep a diary of when any symptoms occur. Then, both records are analyzed to determine if you do have an arrhythmia, whether it is serious, and what measures, if any, should be taken to treat it.

Loop recorders: These recorders are useful for diagnosing arrhythmias that occur infrequently, such as once a month or so. The Endless Loop Recorder is worn continually, but it can be removed to sleep or shower and then easily reattached. It is manually stopped when the arrhythmia has been recorded. The Reveal® Insertable Loop Recorder, about the size of a cigarette lighter, is surgically implanted under the skin, and surgically removed when it is no longer needed, by means of a small incision made under local anesthesia. It can remain in place for months until an irregular heartbeat episode occurs.

Transtelephonic monitor (TTM): Also known as an event recorder, this device is about the size of a small stack of cards. When held in contact with your chest wall, it records your heartbeat, creating an EKG reading, which you can then transmit over the phone to a medical professional, who can interpret it and contact a physician immediately if necessary.

Electrophysiologic Study (EPS)

If your doctor suspects you have, or at are high risk for developing, a serious type of rhythm disturbance, you may undergo an electrophysiologic study (EPS). Wires are threaded inside your heart to stimulate it electrically, in the hope of reproducing the arrhythmia, in order to determine the cause and pinpoint the location. Medications can also be administered during the test to see which control it. Increasingly more frequently today, sound

Chapter Four

wave energy is delivered via a special catheter to a very tiny portion of the heart or electrical system to "destroy" an area responsible for the arrhythmia.

Since this test and therapy are not without risk, they are performed only when there is concern you might develop a life-threatening arrhythmia, or in some cases where the rhythm problem is potentially dangerous, disabling, and resistant to other types of treatment.

Pulmonary Function Tests

Shortness of breath can occur following a heart attack, so this test is used to determine whether it is caused by congestive heart failure or by lung disease. There are two general types of pulmonary function tests: arterial blood gas studies and ventilation tests.

An *arterial blood gas study* is basically a blood test in which blood is drawn from your wrist (because your radial artery is small, easily accessible, and easy to control bleeding from) and sent to a laboratory, where tests are done to check on the amount of various gasses your blood contains. The results show how well your lungs are performing their main task of infusing your blood with oxygen and removing carbon dioxide.

For a *ventilation test*, you are seated and clips are placed over your nose. As you breathe, a test is performed to measure certain components and make sure you are able to breathe efficiently.

A newer type of test to help differentiate a cardiac from pulmonary cause of shortness of breath is a *pulmonary stress test*. Like a cardiac stress test, this involves walking on a treadmill; unlike a cardiac stress test, however, cardiac imaging is not performed. Instead, a specific assessment of lung function is made while you are on the treadmill and helps to determine the main cause of your breathing problem.

KEEPING TRACK OF YOUR TESTS

Now that you know which tests may be ordered, it's important that you keep track of them, so you know which questions to ask and so you can keep track of the results. Being informed empowers you to take control of your recovery. On the next page there is a sample of a diary or journal you can keep.

TREATING THE HEART ATTACK

Today's heart attack treatments are vastly different from those used in the past. Years ago, although there were things that could be done to help someone survive a heart attack, nothing stopped the damage done. Today, this is no longer true. Nowadays, effective heart attack treatments reduce the amount of damage to the heart muscle. These methods include drug therapy, angioplasty, and coronary artery bypass surgery. Here's a rundown on how each works.

Drug Therapy

Clot-busting drugs are used in a procedure called "intravenous thrombolysis." The drug dissolves the blood clot that is causing the heart attack, thus restoring the flow of blood quickly to the heart. These miraculous drugs are most effective when administered within six hours after the heart attack begins—the sooner

MY DIAGNOSTIC TEST DIARY

My In-Hospital Tests

1. Name of the test _____

Result: Normal _____   Abnormal _____

Details _____

What should be done now? _____

Follow-up Testing? _____

Other Instructions _____

2. Name of the test _____

Result: Normal _____   Abnormal _____

Details _____

What should be done now? _____

Follow-up Testing? _____

Other Instructions _____

3. Name of the test _____

Result: Normal _____   Abnormal _____

Details _____

What should be done now? _____

Follow-up Testing? _____

Other Instructions _____

My Follow-up Tests

Name of the test? _____

The reason for the test? _____

When and where is the test? _____

What preparations do I need to make? _____

Can I continue my normal medication?

Yes _____ No _____ Some _____

How long will the test take? _____

Should someone accompany me? _____

If so, who? _____

Should someone drive me home? _____

If so, who? _____

Other special instructions? _____

the better—although they can sometimes be effective after a longer time has elapsed.

There are two different types of clot-busters: tissue plasminogen activator (tPA or TPA) and its related versions, and streptokinase. If you're given a clot-buster, take note of the type you receive. You should generally not be given streptokinase again if you've been given it during a heart attack before, because using streptokinase may potentially cause a severe allergic reaction. So, in the case of a second heart attack, tPA or another clot dissolver would be used.

Angioplasty

Angioplasty (percutaneous transluminal coronary angioplasty, or PTCA) is a procedure that uses a tiny device, usually a balloon, to widen blocked arteries. It has become the most commonly used procedure to restore blood flow to the coronary arteries. The procedure is considered relatively safe and can be performed on people even in their 90s. As the popularity of angioplasty has grown, it has replaced the need for some bypass surgery in many individuals. With angioplasty, recovery is much shorter and less painful.

Although both angioplasty and bypass surgery are considered quite safe, the death rate for angioplasty is lower—less than 1 percent, compared to 1 to 2 percent for bypass surgery. But there are still indications when coronary artery bypass surgery is the preferred treatment.

Angioplasty was once considered riskier for women because, when the technique was first developed (on men), the balloons used were too large for a woman's smaller arteries. Today, smaller catheters and balloons are used.

Chapter Four

Sometimes, a clot-buster is given immediately, and then the woman undergoes catheterization and angioplasty. This is referred to as "facilitated angioplasty." It is done to try to save heart muscle from dying in the situation where there will be a slight delay before emergency angioplasty is performed, even if the delay is relatively short. The idea is that the thrombolytic drug may open up the artery before angioplasty is performed, thereby eliminating the need for emergency PTCA. Whether or not this is beneficial is being researched.

Despite its popularity, emergency angioplasty is not as widely performed as it could be. The demand for this procedure has outstripped the number of facilities where it can be performed. Angioplasty historically can be performed only in hospitals that are equipped to perform open-heart surgery in the rare event that the angioplasty fails and such an operation is needed; most small hospitals do not have these facilities. In this case, patients must be taken to a larger hospital. This has been found to be safe, as long as the procedure can be performed within 90 minutes. More recently, hospitals are being approved to perform "unsupported" emergency angioplasty, wherein the angioplasty procedure is performed and the person is transferred to another institution in the rare situation where a complication occurs and the patient requires emergency cardiac surgery.

The Angioplasty Procedure

During a balloon angioplasty, the patient is given a sedative but remains conscious. The doctor inserts a catheter with a deflated balloon at its tip into the narrowed part of the artery through the groin or arm. Once it is inside the artery, it is maneuvered to the site of the clot. Then, the balloon is inflated, compressing the blood clot and enlarging the inner diameter of the vessel so the blood can once again flow easily. The catheter may also carry a stent, a tiny metallic scaffolding device, which is inserted to keep the artery walls open. This is done to prevent restenosis, which occurs if the tissue within the blood vessel regrows, causing the artery to become narrow again. This is a major problem with angioplasty and is why stents are now used in 80–90 percent of angioplasty procedures. (Stents are discussed more fully later in this chapter.)

After undergoing angioplasty, people often complained about having to lie still for 6–8 hours after the procedure while a 5–10 pound pressure pack was applied to their groin to stop the bleeding. More often nowadays, though, a plug-like device is inserted directly into the artery, which decreases the risk of bleeding.

Angioplasty can be done immediately as an emergency heart attack treatment, or later on, as an elective procedure. Once you're home (a day or two after the procedure), your doctor will probably tell you not to drive or lift anything heavy for a few days. You probably won't have any other restrictions, but you may want to rest for a few days. You can return to work almost immediately, unless your job requires bending or lifting, in which case you'll be told to stay home a few days longer. You'll probably be prescribed a blood-thinning drug, such as clopidogrel (Plavix), which is an anti-clotting drug that you'll stay on for a period ranging from several months to more than a year. Recently, it's been found that, in rare patients, a blood clot may develop at the site of a medication-coated stent when the clopidogrel is discontinued, so many doctors now continue it for longer than one year, and even indefinitely in some cases. You'll also be instructed to take aspirin and probably a cholesterol-lowering statin drug as well.

Chapter Four

In about four to six weeks, your doctor will most likely have you return for an exercise stress test, to make sure your arteries have remained open. He or she will also, hopefully, write an exercise prescription for you, so you can continue (or begin) an exercise program, either at home or in a cardiac rehabilitation program. This "prescription" is actually a program for you to follow so that exercise can help you regain optimum heart health.

Catherine had an angioplasty a few days after her heart attack. "I was given a sedative but, except for that, I was wide-awake" she recounts. "There were machines hovering over my face and chest, so I couldn't see anything. I could talk to the cardiologist, although the sedative made me a little sleepy." So Catherine was awake when the catheter was inserted into the artery in her groin and was guided toward her heart. "When they actually inflated the balloon, I felt some pain, and a little sweaty," Catherine recalls. "When they brought me back to my room. I had to lie flat on my back, but my husband was there, and he fed me lunch. By 9 p.m., the nurse told me to get out of bed, so I walked up and down with my IV. I was walking gingerly, but it felt wonderful to be up and around. After spending another day in the hospital, I went home."

How Successful Is Angioplasty?

Angioplasty can often achieve lasting results. However, arteries can sometimes become narrowed again in the same location, a problem called restenosis, which causes the blood vessel to narrow again. This occurs because the body may generate tissue in a misguided attempt to repair itself, because it misconstrues the angioplasty as an injury.

Restenosis occurs 15 to 40 percent of the time in the three months following the procedure. Although a restenosis rate of up to 40 percent can seem high, it doesn't deter doctors from recommending angioplasty once, or suggesting it be repeated even if restenosis reoccurs, because angioplasty is such an effective procedure and so much less invasive and traumatic than bypass surgery. It's not known why restenosis occurs, but it is more common in people with high blood pressure or diabetes, or who have chest pain due to unstable angina or vasospastic angina, chest pain caused by cardiac spasms, or kidney disease requiring dialysis. Since restenosis is more likely to occur in people with diabetes, they may be more likely to have bypass surgery instead. However, there are a number of ways being developed to try to prevent restenosis, so if you have diabetes and need revascularization, your doctor may decide to try angioplasty at least once and deal with restenosis when and if it happens, rather than have you undergo bypass surgery.

The Use of Stents

Stents were developed to prevent restenosis, but they didn't completely solve this problem. So a new type of stent coated with medication to prevent the tissue from regrowing was developed. As noted earlier, people who receive stents are usually put on anti-clotting medication. In rare cases, a blood clot may develop at the site of the coated stent when the drug is discontinued, so many doctors now continue the medication for longer than one year, and even indefinitely in some cases.

"Intracoronary radiation" is another method used to try to prevent restenosis. This method involves using radiation on the inside of the coronary artery to prevent tissue regrowth, but this is being supplanted by the use of coated stents.

Chapter Four

If you've already had an angioplasty and restenosis occurs, you may need to undergo another angioplasty. This can happen no matter how good a job the doctor did, or how good a patient you were. Don't be discouraged, as the next time the angioplasty may work.

Clot-busters Versus Angioplasty

Just a few years ago, it was assumed that clot-busting drugs would be the best way to eliminate heart-attack-causing blood clots, but this has not been the case. Currently, clot-busting drugs are used frequently, because they can be administered at any size hospital, whereas only larger facilities are equipped to perform angioplasty. However, the success rate for angioplasty is about 95 percent, while it is 70–75 percent for clot-busters. So, the type of treatment you are given during your heart attack emergency will depend on your particular needs, as well as the procedure that is most commonly performed at the hospital where you are taken. It is becoming more common for smaller hospitals to offer emergency angioplasty or, if they do not, to transfer you to a nearby, larger facility for emergency angioplasty in preference to administering thrombolytic drug therapy.

When it comes to clot-busters, the most worrisome complication is bleeding. Basically, clot-busters are blood thinners. Bleeding from them can occur anywhere, including under the skin, the intravenous sites where the drug is injected, the abdomen (if you've had an ulcer), and most worrisome of all, in the brain, which causes a stroke. The risk for this occurring increases with age, so clot-busters are not often used in people over the age of 70.

What Happens in the Hospital

Another problem is that the heart-attack-causing blood clot generally forms in an artery that has been narrowed by coronary heart disease. Even if the clot is dissolved, the narrowed artery remains, and it may become clogged again almost immediately. So, in some cases, the clot-buster may simply turn back the clock a few hours, to right before you had the heart attack, but the conditions for clot formation remain the same. This is not the case with angioplasty. With angioplasty, the artery is reopened and generally stays that way, at least for a while.

Coronary Artery Bypass Surgery

Most of the time, the clot causing the heart attack is dissolved or shrunk as quickly as possible, using either a clot-busting drug or angioplasty. In some cases, though, coronary artery bypass surgery is necessary, either quite soon following a heart attack, perhaps the next day, or later on, depending on the individual.

Although bypass surgery is often referred to as "open-heart surgery," it does not actually require opening the heart. The surgery is performed on the coronary arteries, which lie on the outside surface of the heart. But it does involve using a vein or artery from your body and grafting it onto the vessels of your heart. This grafted vessel provides an alternative route for blood to reach the heart muscle, literally providing a "bypass" around a clogged vessel, which has been narrowed by coronary disease. Despite the growing popularity of angioplasty, bypass surgery remains a very commonly done procedure and can be a lifesaver when angioplasty is not advisable or has failed.

The terminology related to bypass surgery is often misconstrued. For example, people may think a "quadruple" bypass is

Chapter Four

more serious than a "triple" one. That isn't necessarily the case. It is true that the more the number of bypass grafts, the greater was the number of severe narrowings. But the underlying disease process—atherosclerosis—is the same.

Although coronary bypass surgery is considered, by and large, to be a safe procedure, women used to have double the death rate of men. This was mostly due to their smaller coronary arteries, which made the surgery more difficult. Thanks to advances in technology and improved surgical techniques, this has changed, and most current studies find little difference.

Ever since bypasses began being performed, the question of which patients benefit most from the procedure has been hotly debated. Generally, bypass surgery is reserved for patients whose coronary heart disease cannot be adequately treated by clot-busting medication or angioplasty. For instance, your heart's left main artery is a crucial one, since it supplies most of the blood to the main portion of your heart. If that artery becomes critically narrowed, an angioplasty may not be recommended because, if a complication occurred during the procedure, the results could be dangerous.

Also, women who suffer from severe chest pain due to coronary artery disease that can't be relieved by medication or an angioplasty may be referred for bypass surgery. Bypass surgery may also be the procedure for people who have undergone angioplasty repeatedly but whose vessels closed up again, or for those who underwent bypass surgery years ago but whose grafts have now become clogged. Bypass surgery is also used for people who have both clogged arteries and a heart valve problem that needs to be surgically repaired at the same time.

The Coronary Artery Bypass Procedure

Although there have been improvements, the basics of coronary artery bypass surgery have not changed in the last three decades since its invention. The bypass procedure uses veins or arteries taken from your own body—usually either the saphenous vein in the leg, the internal mammary artery (also called the internal thoracic artery) in the chest, or more recently, the radial artery in the forearm. The vein or artery is then grafted onto the surface of the heart. Since more than one graft is usually made, a combination of these vessels is often used.

The surgery is done using general anesthesia. If the bypass is to be done with your leg vein, that vein is removed after you are put to sleep. Then the surgeon makes an opening in your aorta, which is your main artery, and another in the narrowed artery beyond the blockage. The surgeon than sews one end of the grafted vein to each opening, creating a new route along which the blood from your aorta can flow. If the surgeon is using your internal mammary artery, the end where it originates is left in place and the remainder is repositioned and inserted below the blockage in the affected artery, thereby creating the bypass.

Minimally Invasive Coronary Bypass Surgery

In the past few years, there have been some changes made in hopes of creating a way in which to accomplish the same goals of restoring blood flow to the heart without the major type of surgery that traditional bypass surgery requires. This new approach is known as minimally invasive coronary bypass surgery.

Chapter Four

However, traditional surgery still makes up the vast majority of bypass operations.

During "beating heart," or minimally invasive bypass surgery, the surgeon performs the surgery through a small incision in the chest of about 3 inches (a 6–8 inch incision down the chest is used for traditional coronary bypass surgery). Then, using specialized equipment to hold and stabilize the heart, the surgeon performs the procedure while the heart is still beating. This type of surgery is not suitable for all types of cases; it is most easily performed when a single vessel (left anterior descending or right coronary artery) needs to be bypassed.

"Port access surgery" is another type of minimally invasive coronary bypass surgery. This type of surgery is used when more than one coronary artery needs to be bypassed. In this case, the heart is stopped, and the patient is connected to a heart-lung machine by a tube placed in the groin and threaded to the femoral artery. The heart-lung machine allows for the circulation of the blood throughout the body while the surgeon performs the bypass. This procedure eliminates the need for the large chest incision ordinarily performed during bypass surgery, resulting in a shorter recovery time.

Much less commonly used today, but growing in availability and popularity, is coronary surgery using a robot! The surgeon sits in the operating room next to a computer console 10–20 feet from where you are lying on the operating table. The surgeon remotely controls the robot, which can perform surgery through approximately four small (⅓ inch) puncture wounds in your chest rather than through a large incision. Because the robot uses metal sticks, the incision can be smaller than what would be needed for a surgeon's hands. This smaller incision further minimizes pain and recovery time.

Although minimally invasive coronary bypass surgery sounds good, this type of surgery is not for everyone. Your surgeon must consider the location and extent of your coronary artery disease, among other factors, in deciding whether or not to offer these newer approaches.

FIVE
―――
On the Road to Recovery

Hospital stays for an uncomplicated heart attack used to stretch for weeks but are now squeezed into only a few days. Your stay may be the shortest if you've undergone angioplasty. This is because the procedure makes certain that your coronary arteries are open. You may spend a few days longer if you received a clot-buster drug, because your doctor will want to be certain your symptoms don't return. But even if you've undergone bypass surgery—which is major surgery—this may not even guarantee you a week of hospitalization.

GETTING READY FOR DISCHARGE

Even before you are discharged from the hospital, there are steps you can take to transition yourself to the healthier lifestyle that awaits you once you get home. Much of this preparation used to take place while you were in the hospital, but no longer. It used to be standard for a woman who had experienced a heart attack to be hospitalized for three weeks. There was plenty of time to go over medications and diet and exercise plans, and also to really absorb the significance of what had happened. But that three-week stay has dwindled now to just days. Too often, heart attack survivors are discharged while they are still trying to come to grips with the idea that they had a heart attack!

This is unfortunate, because it's only natural that, if you've just had a heart attack, you may suddenly become more receptive to making difficult lifestyle changes. With time, you may lose sight of the gravity of what you experienced. Don't fall into that trap. Your long-term survival and quality of life depend on the positive changes you make. The sooner the better.

Your Discharge Diary

To help fill in the gap between the hospital and home, the American Heart Association instituted a program called "Get With the Guidelines." This program is designed to ensure you have all the basic information you need before you are discharged. But if your hospital doesn't have this program or a similar one, don't worry. Here's the information you need to accomplish the same thing.

Get a loose-leaf notebook or a spiral notebook divided into different sections, and keep it handy. Start using it to compile information now, before you leave the hospital. You can also take it with you when you go to your doctor for your follow-up visit. This will help start your recuperation on a positive note and remind you of important facts you may forget later. One component of your notebook will be the "Information to Get Before You're Discharged" questionnaire provided below. Some of the answers needed for the questionnaire you may not have now, so you can fill them in later. As you continue reading this book, we'll also give you plenty of suggestions and tips about controlling

On the Road to Recovery

blood pressure, cholesterol, and the like, which you can keep a record of in your notebook.

Look over the questionnaire below. If you do not have the answers to the questions regarding your hospital treatment, call your doctor and get the details. Take charge of your health, starting right now. Know and understand exactly what happened to your body; it's important because it will guide you toward a full recovery. Become informed. Take charge of your recovery!

Many of these topics are covered in depth in subsequent chapters. But this is the personal information you need to know as a baseline, so you know where you stand as you get started on a healthier lifestyle.

Information to Get Before You're Discharged

If you're already home and you don't have this information, take this list to your next doctor's appointment and get the information. Or call your doctor's office and ask how you can get it.

1. Start your notebook with hospital information. What procedures did you have while you were hospitalized?

- Were you treated with a clot-busting drug?
  If so, which one? _____
- Did you undergo a coronary angiogram (also known as coronary catheterization)?
  Yes _____ No _____
  What did the angiogram show?
- Did you undergo an angioplasty?
  Yes _____ No _____

Chapter Five

- If so, was a stent used?
  Yes _____ No _____
  If yes, what type? _____
  How many? _____
  Where _____
- Were any narrow areas of the coronary arteries left
  untreated? Yes _____ No _____
  If so, which? _____

2. Start a new page with doctor and appointment information.
Who is your doctor?

_____

This is not a trick question. Many doctors may have seen you
when you were hospitalized. Will the cardiologist who saw you in
the hospital provide your follow-up care? Will he or she be your
regular doctor?

My follow-up appointments are

_____

3. The next section will be used to keep track of your heart medications.
Keep track of which medications you take now. Know which drugs
you are supposed to take. For prescription drugs, be sure to note
the brand names or the generic names, and the exact strengths in
which they are prescribed. Also include any special instructions,
such as how the drugs should be taken (with food, for example)
and whether they should be taken for a specified time or indefinitely. Note also whether you are supposed to take the whole pill,
or just half. Also specify any that require follow-up tests. Keep this
listing up to date.

On the Road to Recovery

The following drugs are now considered to be the standard for preventing another heart attack. If you are not on these four types of drugs, you should ask your doctor for the reason.

_____ An aspirin or aspirin-type drug, such as Plavix, or both

_____ A beta blocker

_____ A cholesterol-lowering drug

_____ An ACE inhibitor

You also may be prescribed nitroglycerin, for long-term use or for use in an emergency if you have chest pain. Make sure you know how to use it, including how it should be taken during an emergency.

Start a new page in the medications section to help you keep track of other medications you take. Here's a sample format you can use to help you keep track of the medications you take, both prescription and over the counter:

My first medication is: _____

I take it _____ times a day at _____

I take it because _____

I will be taking it for (fill in a specific period of time) or indefinitely.

My second medication is: _____

I take it _____ times a day at _____

I take it for _____

I will be taking it for (fill in a specific period of time) or indefinitely.

Chapter Five

You can use this format for whatever number of medications you take.

4. The next section is about restrictions.

List all restrictions you may have and the dates your doctor says you can resume your usual activities. Restrictions can depend on your heart attack recovery, any complications you may have developed due to your heart attack, and any complications from procedures you had in the hospital. Restrictions can be very short-term, such as whether or not you can bathe and when. Or they can be for the duration of your recuperation, affecting such things as driving, lifting heavy objects, sports, or sexual activity.

I can resume driving (fill in when) _____

I can resume lifting objects such as a bag of groceries _____

I can resume exercising _____

I can resume my favorite sports _____

I can resume sexual activity _____

5. The next section is for emergency instructions. Put a sticky tab on this section and be sure others know about it, too—just in case.

In an emergency situation, this is the number I should call (generally 911): _____

My doctor's emergency telephone number: _____

Who in my family knows CPR? _____

Who in my workplace knows CPR? _____

Is there a cardiac defibrillator where I work? _____
At home? _____

If not, whom at work should I discuss this with? _____

On the Road to Recovery

NOW YOU'RE ON THE MEND

If you have a career or juggle a busy family life—or both—you'll be wondering how much you'll be able to do once you get home. Generally, how you feel will dictate the amount of activity you do, and the intensity with which you do it.

"Just a few weeks before I had my heart attack," Alison recalls, "I'd been joking with a friend that I needed a maternity leave—without a baby—just to catch up with my projects. Suddenly my wish was answered, in a way. The heart attack gave me the time off I needed, but I didn't have the energy to do any of those projects I'd planned. In fact, I remember taking slow walks with the dog and sitting for hours on the front porch swing for the six weeks I stayed at home."

Regaining Strength

This is your first priority. Before you even think of resuming your regular activities, you'll have to slowly regain your strength and stamina. You may be surprised to find out how much energy even small tasks take. Don't despair. It will all come back to you. Each day you'll get stronger. Recovery time is time well spent.

Immediately upon returning home from the hospital, you may feel suddenly fragile and doubt the wisdom of the decision to discharge you. Bear in mind, though, that while you were in the hospital, you were able to walk around your room, and up and down the halls, at a slow, comfortable pace. Take time the first week to become accustomed to being at home. Expect to be tired, and realize that you probably won't feel like doing what you were doing before. Don't worry; you're going to eventually be back to living a fully normal, active life. Your energy will return gradually, over a period of several weeks.

Chapter Five

RETURNING TO NORMALCY

A heart attack can pack an emotional wallop. Although sometimes surviving a heart attack can bring with it a powerful sense of relief, this is not necessarily true for many women. Many suffer with anxiety, depression, and loneliness.

"My heart attack was much more hard for me to get over emotionally than it was physically," Carol observes. "I was never sick a day in my life before I had my heart attack. I'd never been in pain. The hardest thing about dealing with this was the head game, or knowing this actually happened and that it was something that I had no control over. I go to sleep and I remember the blackness. This has been very hard for me to handle."

According to Alison, "The hardest thing is getting used to the idea that I'm going to die someday. That feeling—my husband always said I had lived like I was immortal and, after my heart attack, I didn't have that feeling anymore."

Anne says, "I went through heart surgery and focused on the physical aspect of it. All of my cardiologists seemed to take for granted I was fine. It wasn't until months later when a cardiologist, who happened to be a friend, looked me in the eye and said, 'Well, how are you doing emotionally?' that it hit me, and I burst into tears."

DEALING WITH YOUR EMOTIONS

Men more commonly suffer their heart attacks earlier in life than women do, and men are more likely to be married, with a wife to serve as an emotional buffer. Women are more likely to be older and possibly widowed by the time of their heart attack. Their children may be grown and living away from home, and they may

On the Road to Recovery

be socially isolated. If you feel lonely or isolated, talk to your doctor about it, join a cardiac rehab program to meet other heart attack survivors, or see if your hospital has a "heart club" for survivors. There are also more and more organizations getting underway to help women heart attack survivors meet and support each other. See the Resources section in this book.

Dealing with Anxiety and Depression

Until recently, there was no organized support system for women heart attack survivors. Increasingly, there is some help offered, but such programs are still in their infancy. This is a problem, when you consider that a heart attack can raise serious emotional issues, such as:

- Sudden recognition of mortality that comes from experiencing a life-threatening illness
- Concern over how others will see you, especially if you were apparently healthy before and your heart attack occurred suddenly
- The need to fit recuperation into what may already be a very busy life
- Making major lifestyle changes, such as quitting smoking, changing the way you eat, or having to exercise
- Dealing with medical bills and other financial issues

It's no wonder that women report high levels of both anxiety and depression following a heart attack. Anxiety is defined as a vague, unpleasant emotion that is experienced in anticipation of some (usually ill-defined) event. But for many women, there is nothing vague about the sense of discomfort, jumpiness, and

Chapter Five

nervousness they find themselves dealing with following their heart attack.

"I'm a very independent person," says Carol. "I do my own thing; my husband does his. But this has been very hard for me to handle. I'm so used to getting in the car and just going without a thought, but after my heart attack, the first time I went to buy some quilting fabric, I was scared. I had to make myself go on my own."

Depression is also a major problem, but it's rare that a woman is asked about her emotional state. Instead, the depression that too often accompanies a heart attack is also too often misdiagnosed or inappropriately treated. Certainly, some sadness or worry is normal after a heart attack or heart surgery, so it can be difficult to distinguish between clinical depression and a sense of normal sadness or concern that may accompany recovery. But here is a rundown on symptoms that could indicate depression may not lift:

- Having a depressed mood for most of the day
- Loss of interest or pleasure in almost all activities most of the day
- Significant weight loss or gain or an increase or decrease in appetite
- Insomnia or excessive sleepiness
- Restlessness
- Fatigue or loss of energy
- Feelings of worthlessness or excessive or inappropriate guilt
- Diminished ability to think or concentrate, or indecisiveness

- Recurring thoughts of death or of suicide, a suicide attempt, or a specific plan for committing suicide

If you experience any of these and you cannot shake free of them, you should discuss them with your doctor, social worker, or other appropriate individual who can arrange for you to get help.

There are numerous treatments for depression, including individual and group therapy and treatment with antidepressants. Some of these medications, particularly the older types, can produce such side effects as high blood pressure, low blood pressure, and heartbeat irregularities. This doesn't mean that the medications cannot be safely used, but your doctor should consider the type and severity of your heart disease, any adverse side effects the medications may have, and their demonstrated safety record on people with heart disease before selecting the medication that is right for you.

Stress Relief

When asked what they believe caused their heart attack, women will often answer "stress." This is not an uncommon response; it's apt to come up, even if a woman smokes, is diabetic, or has a sky-high cholesterol level. So is stress the culprit?

There isn't enough research evidence to link stress to heart attacks in the same way as such major risk factors as high cholesterol, diabetes, or smoking. Still, there is enough evidence to consider stress as a suspect contributing cause. But whether stress is a major culprit or not, being "under stress" can certainly lead one to engage in unhealthy activities, such as smoking, drinking heavily, or eating too much. Also, it's well known that tremendous stress can have an impact on the heart. This can be seen in the

Chapter Five

increased rate of heart attacks when an earthquake strikes, for instance. All this makes the goal of stress reduction worthwhile.

What Is Stress?

Simply put, stress is our body's response to the perception of threat. As we have evolved over millions of years, such a response was essential to survival. This is known as the "flight or fight" syndrome. In modern times, this response may still have value, if you are directly threatened with being mugged, for example. But the feeling of stress, along with its accompanying emotions of anger and hostility, is too often triggered by the tiny annoyances of everyday life.

Also, not all stress is bad stress. Positive stress can be associated with joy, exhilaration, and a feeling of a job well done.

Although stress is an emotion that you usually "feel" consciously, your response to it activates mechanisms within your body of which you may not be aware. When faced with a stressful situation, your autonomic nervous system responds by increasing production of such chemicals as cortisol and epinephrine, which increases the heart rate, raises the blood pressure, and speeds up the metabolism. Stress has implications for coronary artery disease as well; stress can make the blood more likely to clot, which can increase heart attack risk.

Changing the way you deal with stress can be as difficult as giving up smoking, or learning not to reach for a cookie when something goes amiss. But there are ways to make stress more manageable. Here are some suggestions:

- *Meditation:* Meditation is a process in which one tries to achieve awareness. There are different types of

On the Road to Recovery

meditation. Transcendental meditation (TM), teaches practitioners to focus on a single object, or a short phrase called a mantra. On the other hand, practitioners of "mindfulness" meditation learn to pay close moment-to-moment attention to achieve awareness. Practitioners find this an excellent way not only to reduce stress but also to eliminate unnecessary worrying.

- *Yoga:* A system of Hindu philosophy and religion, yoga combines relaxation, deep breathing, meditation, and stretching. *Hatha-yoga*, the most familiar type, employs a series of poses, known as *asanas*, along with a special breathing technique. These exercises maintain flexibility and teach physical and mental control. By using breathing, yoga practitioners also are encouraged to clear their mind and slow their thoughts, features shared by adherents to meditation. *Pilates*, another form of yoga, is a system of strengthening and stretching exercises designed to develop the body's core muscles (abdominal, low back, hips, and gluteals). There's even a blend called "Yogilates."

- *Biofeedback:* Biofeedback teaches you how to control bodily functions that are usually considered involuntary, including skin temperature, muscle contraction, heart rate, blood pressure, and brain waves. Practicing biofeedback has been found to be helpful in easing chest pain and the vascular pain from diabetes, and in lowering high blood pressure. Biofeedback is often combined with other, more general relaxation techniques.

- *Relaxation techniques:* These are methods in which you consciously release your muscular tension to achieve a state of mental calm. Active relaxation consists of alternatively tensing and relaxing all of the muscles in your body. Passive relaxation involves clearing the mind to concentrate on a single phrase or sound.

- *Virtual vacation:* For most of us, it's impossible to take frequent long vacations. But, using only your imagination, you can take frequent "mini-vacations." This is done via a technique called visualization, a fancy name for what used to be called simply "daydreaming." Close your eyes and imagine your favorite vacation spot. Is it the beach? You can see yourself lying there. Isn't the sun warm? Or perhaps you're flying down your favorite ski slope. Can't you feel the fresh, cool air on your face? Or can't you see your hair fly as you sail along in your boat? Even just a five-minute virtual vacation can leave you feeling surprisingly refreshed.

- *Pampering yourself:* Sometimes in our stress-filled days it's easy to cram in too much and neglect being good to yourself. Treat yourself to a quiet hour with a good book, see a movie, or take a long bubble bath.

HOME AND FAMILY LIFE

If there are younger children at home, you're going to need help. If you're married and your husband can take a week or two off from work, this might be an ideal solution. If not, hire outside help if you can afford to, or expand your babysitter's hours.

Here are some general instructions on what you will be able to do. Your doctor may give you more specifics tailored to your own health. When you first get home, feel free to walk around the house. If you live in a two-level house, you can climb the stairs as often as you wish, as long as you don't become tired. You may find that you need to climb the steps slowly at first. You can also do the simple housekeeping chores you usually do, as long as you don't overdo. Perhaps you're accustomed to doing two loads of laundry each week and keeping the floors buffed and your carpets lint-free. The cleanliness police are not going to be summoned if you do the laundry less often or a few dust bunnies collect in the corner.

This is the time to lean on your family for support. If they are accustomed to having you run the house, establish some new rules. Your family will need to share in the workload while you recover, but you may need to make these changes permanent if you were overburdened before.

You can lift a baby, but don't plan on hoisting a toddler for a while. You can participate in the school activities you're accustomed to doing, such as attending school plays, concerts, parent-child conferences, and attending to other familial duties. If you shoulder the responsibility of caring for aging parents, you'll need help in this as well, so don't feel shy about calling upon family members to do their part. Consider enlisting the help of social service agencies as well. The social worker at your hospital may be able to advise you.

Bear in mind that you've had a heart attack. That's serious business, and you have a responsibility to look out for your own health.

Getting Back Behind the Wheel

Driving is a part of modern life. You're most likely accustomed to spending at least part of your day behind the wheel, either shuttling your kids back and forth to their activities, or going to your job, or both. After your heart attack, you won't be able to drive for a while, but how long this restriction will last depends on your individual case. If your heart attack was uncomplicated, or you underwent angioplasty, your doctor may want you to avoid driving for one to two weeks. This is mostly to guard against your becoming stressed in the event you are involved in an accident, as well as to allow your groin to heal after the cardiac catheterization and angioplasty. If you absolutely must get back on the road, you may be able to convince your doctor to allow you to drive sooner. Remember, though, safeguarding your health is the most important thing. If you've had coronary artery bypass surgery, this nondriving period will definitely be longer, about four to six weeks, so your chest can heal from the surgery.

Sports and Exercise

If you're a fitness buff or enjoy athletic sports, like tennis or golf, you should be able to eventually return to your normal activities without any restrictions. How long this takes depends on the severity of the heart attack and the activity. Generally, you can return to your usual athletic activities after about a month.

Enjoying Sex

Soon after a heart attack, anything that entails physical stress—even something as enjoyable as sex—can be scary. Unfortunately, women are very unlikely to discuss this problem with their doctor—especially if their doctor is male. But even women who see female cardiologists may be reluctant to raise the issue, especially if they belong to an older generation.

Male heart attack survivors encounter problems with sex. In fact, it's very common. Erectile dysfunction, or impotence, is a

On the Road to Recovery

common byproduct of coronary heart disease. In fact, impotence may be a sign of undiagnosed heart disease in a man, because the penis requires an adequate blood supply to have and maintain an erection. But, although signs of sexual dysfunction can be less obvious in women, they can be no less stressful. Loss of sexual desire, anxiety about sexual activity causing another heart attack, and inability to achieve orgasm can be common problems.

It doesn't have to be that way. The key to a good sexual relationship is the same as the key to any other good relationship: communication. The couple that is accustomed to discussing their problems frankly can often find it easy to iron out differences in the sexual arena once the topic is broached. But sexual dysfunction can have medical causes, which can be solved only with the help of your doctor. So, even if the subject of sex usually leaves you tongue-tied or blushing, talk to your doctor. After a few words, your doctor should be able to pick up the conversational ball. Unfortunately, though, some doctors are not very good at discussing sex. If this is the case, it often helps to be as specific as possible about your concern.

Loss of sexual desire is the most common problem a woman experiences after a heart attack. This can be due to depression. Your self-image may have changed; you may feel less vital, or more fragile. If you had coronary bypass surgery, you may take a while to heal, or you may be left with a surgical scar that can make you self-conscious. You may be experiencing sexual difficulties that are more due to age, such as vaginal dryness, which may accompany menopause. In this case, a good lubricant may be effective. You may be taking certain cardiovascular drugs that dampen sexual arousal or the ability to reach orgasm. In this case, your doctor may be able to substitute other medications.

Chapter Five

One of the biggest fears experienced by both women and men is the worry that sexual excitement will lead to another heart attack. Happily, this fear is more the stuff of novels and movies than of reality.

If you've passed your stress test after a heart attack, your doctor will most likely clear you for having sex. If you can climb a flight of stairs without experiencing cardiac symptoms (like chest pain or shortness of breath), your doctor will probably give you permission to have "passive" sex. This means, basically, that you're on the bottom. Also, having sex with a familiar partner (such as a spouse) generally causes less sexual excitement and is easier to handle.

If you can climb two flights of stairs without experiencing cardiac symptoms, you should be able to handle any type of sexual acrobatics you wish, within the bounds of what is safe for someone who never had a heart attack, of course!

Here are some guidelines that may be helpful:

- Follow your exercise prescription. Regular physical exercise helps you perform any type of physical activity—sex included—with ease.
- Consider switching your sexual encounter from night to mornings when you are more rested.
- Don't engage in sex after eating a big meal or heavy drinking.
- If you experience cardiac symptoms during sex, such as angina, the chest pain that sometimes accompanies heart disease, discuss it with your doctor. You may be advised to take nitroglycerin before sex to lessen such symptoms. Above all, be patient with yourself and your partner.

On the Road to Recovery

- Talk to your doctor, should you need to. A diminished sex drive is not unusual after a heart attack; with time, normalcy should return. If, however, you find this problem becoming cemented into a pattern, you should discuss it with your doctor.

Sex is a healthy, normal part of life, and an activity you should certainly not have to sacrifice to heart disease. In fact, if you strive for the other goals outlined in this book, including quitting smoking, losing weight, and improving your physical condition, you may find yourself enjoying sex more than you have in years!

GOING BACK TO WORK

If your heart attack was mild and you are being treated only with medication, or if you had an angioplasty as well, you may be allowed to return to your job in as little as one to three weeks, depending on how physically demanding your work is. If you underwent bypass surgery, plan on staying home for at least three to four weeks.

If you're the sole breadwinner in your home, or if your job demands it, you may need to get back to work as soon as possible. But, if you have the opportunity to take some time off, this might be the time to take advantage of that. It's sometimes tempting to try to return quickly, to prove to your boss (or to yourself) that you can do everything you did before. Your boss and coworkers may be very understanding at first, but once you're back, they'll expect you to work at your previous capacity. Sometimes it's better to stay home a little longer and come back as your old self rather than return first on a part-time basis.

Chapter Five

This is true if your job is not only physically demanding, but mentally demanding as well. In that case, you might find that your powers of concentration are not as sharp as they were before your heart attack. Your mental prowess will return but, again, this is part of the recuperation process. Karen, a prosecutor, found this out when she was recuperating from her heart attack. When she did go back to work, she eased into it, first working three days a week, then four, and finally a full five-day workweek.

"After my heart attack," Karen says, "I was surprised that my powers of concentration had been impaired. I could read newspapers and magazine articles, but books were beyond me. Because my work requires such concentration and reading, I was reluctant to go back to work. My powers of concentration did come back, but I remember being very troubled by this before they did. It took me about six months to feel like I'd hit my stride again."

Before you hurry back to work, consider that sometimes a heart attack may be a blessing in disguise. This was a pause in your life that you didn't ask for, but you might want to take advantage of the situation. Your emotions may be in turmoil. A heart attack can be a life-changing event, and you may very well need time to emotionally assimilate what happened to you.

WHAT ABOUT PREGNANCY?

By the time most women have their heart attack, they are past menopause. But this is not true of all women. Some heart attack survivors are relatively young and may wish to become pregnant. Pregnancy carries risks even for healthy women, especially those over 35. But the likelihood of most heart attack survivors being able to carry through a successful pregnancy and deliver a healthy baby is greater now than ever before. It all depends on the individual woman—how well her heart functions and is capable of withstanding the rigors of pregnancy and delivery.

Pregnancy and the Normal Heart

Being pregnant produces changes in your body that can challenge the heart, but the vast majority of women take these biological changes in stride. For the damaged heart, however, pregnancy makes the daily workload that much harder. For instance, when you are pregnant, your blood volume increases 40–50 percent by the fifth month. That represents a vast increase in the amount of blood your heart has to pump. Your heart also beats ten to twenty more times per minute than before you were pregnant, contracting more strongly with each beat. During delivery, your heart may be called upon to work four to five times as hard is it did before you were pregnant. If your heart is weak, this can be dangerous. In addition, as your baby grows inside you, it needs more and more oxygen and nutrients. Damage that makes it difficult for your heart to supply enough oxygen to your body will only make your heart struggle harder if it must supply oxygen to your enlarging uterus and developing baby as well. These are all difficult challenges, but with careful management and planning, most heart attack survivors can overcome these and give birth to a healthy baby.

Whether you should become pregnant and how closely you should be monitored by a cardiologist during pregnancy depend on how much damage and what type of damage your heart attack caused. If the damage left you with serious complications, you may need to be closely monitored by a team that includes a cardiologist and an obstetrician very experienced in high-risk pregnancies. If you were not left with what seem to be serious complications but your doctor seems unduly pessimistic, consider seeking a second opinion at a major medical center from a cardiologist who specializes in dealing with high-risk pregnancies. This way, you'll be certain you have an accurate idea of the risks involved to make your decision.

Pregnancy Planning

The best way for a cardiologist to evaluate just how likely it is your heart problem will endanger your pregnancy is with a thorough, up-to-date evaluation of your heart. The ideal time to do this is before you become pregnant. Of course, pregnancy can occur without planning. But if possible, plan ahead.

When you are not pregnant, your doctor has the freedom to perform all the necessary diagnostic tests without any fear of harming an unborn baby. If you are already pregnant, the choice of tests is more limited, but even so, there are a number of tests that can be safely performed, including echocardiography. Your doctor can also check you for any heartbeat irregularities by performing various monitoring tests. Cardiac catheterization, which is done before angioplasty or coronary bypass surgery, involves high-dose radiation. If you needed to undergo this, it could be done, as long as a lead apron shielded your abdomen and pelvis. Your doctor would want to wait until after your first trimester, if possible.

Cardiovascular Drugs During Pregnancy

Taking any medication when you become pregnant becomes an important issue, and cardiovascular drugs are no exception.

On the Road to Recovery

Drugs that pose no safety hazard to you may be dangerous for your unborn child.

To be on the safe side, when you're pregnant, you should take drugs only if they're absolutely needed. But, nowadays, most heart attack survivors take several medications on a daily basis, such as drugs to control high blood pressure, cholesterol, and diabetes, as well as medications specifically for your heart.

The impact of these drugs on your pregnancy also must be considered on an individual basis. If you've discussed your impending pregnancy with your cardiologist beforehand, your doctor will have the opportunity to wean you off any potentially dangerous drugs, or substitute safer drugs for them ahead of time. If you do require medication, many drugs now on the market have established safety records, so your doctor will be able to recommend the right medication for you. But remember, don't assume any drug is safe. Discuss every medication you take (both prescription and over the counter) with your doctor. Bear in mind as well that, if you are taking medications for a heart problem, abruptly stopping can be risky, so contact your doctor immediately.

UNDERSTANDING CARDIOVASCULAR DRUGS

Over the years, cardiac drugs have played an increasingly important role in heart attack prevention. The following drugs are used to prevent heart attacks, lower blood pressure, improve cholesterol balance, and help with the symptoms of congestive heart failure. More medications are coming on the market, so this list is not intended to be all inclusive. But here is a rundown of the major drugs and their types, listed according to alphabetical order. Some drugs have more than one usage, but they are listed in their main category.

ACE Inhibitors

An ACE inhibitor, or angiotension converting enzyme, decreases angiotensin II, a natural chemical in the body that narrows the blood vessels and raises blood pressure. Obviously, ACE inhibitors are important in lowering blood pressure, but they are also used in the treatment of heart failure, where they have been shown to strengthen the heart muscle and prolong life. They are also used to prevent heart attacks and strokes, and they help prevent kidney damage in people with diabetes. Examples of ACE inhibitors include enalapril maleate (Vasotec), lisinopril (Zestril, Prinivil), captopril (Capoten), fosinopril (Monopril), ramipril (Altace), quinapril (Accupril), perindopril (Aceon), trandolapril (Mavik), and moexipril (Univasc). Some of these are available generically.

Angiotensin II Receptor Blockers (ARBs)

These are related to the ACE inhibitors. This is a newer class of high blood pressure medications. They have a slightly different mechanism but have a similar effect on blood vessels. Currently, they are generally prescribed for people who have high blood pressure or heart failure and cannot tolerate an ACE inhibitor, or who have both diabetes and kidney disease. Examples of ARBs include losartan (Cozaar), valsartan (Diovan), irbesartan (Avapro), candesartan (Atacand), and several others.

On the Road to Recovery

Anti-Angina Drugs

Nitroglycerin, which is a form of nitrate, provides temporary relief from chest pain by dilating your blood vessels, effectively enabling more oxygen to reach the heart. It also reduces the workload of your heart.

Nitrates come in various forms. Short-acting nitroglycerin can be used to relieve chest pain during an acute episode of angina (chest pain). It is taken as a small pill under the tongue or as a spray, and it works within five minutes, lasting for 10–30 minutes. Longer-acting nitroglycerin, which can last for several hours, is available as pills, patches, and ointments. It is also used along with other cardiac drugs. Examples of nitrates include Nitrostat, Isordil, Ismo, Imdur, Nitrol-Bid Ointment, Nitro-Dur, and Transderm-Nitro Transdermal. Generic preparations are also available.

Anti-Arrythmic Drugs

Several anti-arrhythmic medications, the type of drugs used most often to treat irregular heartbeats, have been developed over the past few years. Sodium channel blockers, which slowed electrical conduction in the heart, were widely used but are not generally employed anymore; examples of this type of drug are quinidine (Quinidex) and procainamide (Procan). Still being used is a type of anti-arrhythmic drug that slows the heart's electrical impulses by blocking the potassium channels in the heart. Examples include amiodarone, sotalol, and dofetilide.

Beta blockers and calcium channel blockers are also used to treat irregular heartbeats.

Chapter Five

Anti-Clotting Drugs

Aspirin apparently prevents heart attacks by thinning the blood and making it less likely to clot. It is used as a heart attack preventative and is also given to people after angioplasty and coronary bypass surgery. People who believe they may be having a heart attack are told to chew an aspirin to get the drug into their bloodstream more quickly.

Some people cannot take aspirin safely because of adverse side effects. By far the most common side effect is stomach upset. Aspirin can also cause intestinal bleeding, as well as easy skin bruising. People with blood disorders involving their platelets (blood clotting components) are at increased risk if their platelet counts are low. Some people are allergic to aspirin and should, obviously, avoid taking it. Aspirin can also cause tinnitus, or ringing in the ears.

It is also estimated that about one in five people are completely or partially aspirin resistant. Therefore, taking aspirin would have less, or no, effect. A blood test is being developed that will be used to identify these people, so they can be given alternatives.

Clopidogrel (Plavix) is used, alone or in combination with aspirin, to cut the risk of another heart attack. People who have undergone angioplasties with stents were told in the past to take clopidogrel for up to a year to prevent blood clots. They are now increasingly being told to take it for longer than one year, perhaps indefinitely. Plavix may be prescribed to people who have peripheral vascular disease, which is leg pain due to poor circulation, an indication of atherosclerosis in the blood vessels of the legs, which is associated with an increased risk of a heart attack. This condition may be a complication of diabetes.

On the Road to Recovery

Warfarin (Coumadin) is a very powerful blood thinner that interferes with your blood's normal coagulation. Warfarin is commonly prescribed for people whose heart valves have been replaced with mechanical valves, or to prevent stroke in those who suffer from atrial fibrillation, a type of heartbeat irregularity. If you're taking it, your blood must be tested periodically. Your doctor may also give you a list of foods that affect your blood test; you should eat these as you normally would, avoiding limiting or bingeing on them, so they don't affect the test results.

Heparin is another blood thinner used when quick action is needed. It can only be given by injection and used to be only available intravenously. Now another type (low molecular weight heparin) has been developed that is injected subcutaneously but can be given on an outpatient basis, and it doesn't require the multiple blood tests that the intravenous type does.

Thrombin inhibitors form another class of blood thinners currently being developed. Thrombin inhibitors may eventually be available in oral form and will not require blood tests. This will be the next advance in anti-clotting therapy.

Beta Blockers

Beta blockers block the effects of adrenaline, which raises the heart rate and blood pressure. Beta blockers also slow the heart's contractions, reduce its need for oxygen, and decrease the amount of blood the heart must pump. They have been shown to prevent heart attacks, lower blood pressure, help regulate arrhythmia, reduce chest pain, and improve heart failure symptoms. There are many types and brands on the market, including sotalol (Betapace), timolol (Blocadren), esmolol (Brevibloc), carteolol

(Cartrol), carvedilol (Coreg), nadolol (Corgard), propranolol (Inderal, Inderal-LA), betaxolol (Kerlone), penbutolol (Levatol), metoprolol (Lopressor), labetalol (Normodyne, Trandate), acebutolol (Sectral), atenolol (Tenormin), metoprolol succinate (Toprol-XL), pindolol (Visken), and bisoprolol (Zebeta). Some of these are available in generic forms.

Calcium Channel Blockers

Calcium channel blockers slow the rate at which calcium passes into the cell membranes of the heart muscle and into the vessel walls. This relaxes the vessels, enabling the blood to flow through them more easily, and lowering blood pressure. Calcium channel blockers include nifedipine (Adalat, Procardia), verapamil (Calan), nicardipine (Cardene), isradipine (DynaCirc), amlodipine (Lotrel, Norvasc), nimodipine (Nimotop), felodipine (Plendil), and nisoldipine (Sular).

Cholesterol Drugs

Statins are the most popular cholesterol-lowering drugs on the market and are often prescribed for heart attack survivors, even if cholesterol levels are normal. Statins lower LDL cholesterol, the "bad" cholesterol, by 20–60 percent. They also have a modest effect in lowering triglycerides and raising HDL cholesterol, the "good" cholesterol. But the major impact of the statins is on LDL cholesterol, and they lower this type of cholesterol more than any other of the cholesterol-lowering drugs on the market. Statin drugs include lovastatin (Mevacor), simvastatin (Zocor), pravastatin (Pravachol), fluvastatin (Lescol), atorvastatin (Lipitor), and rosuvastatin (Crestor). Generic versions of the first three are available, and more may become available soon.

On the Road to Recovery

Although statins are extremely effective, their effect is not dose dependent: if you double the amount of the statin, you won't get double the reduction in your cholesterol; you'll get much less of a benefit. So, if the statin does not lower your LDL cholesterol enough, or if you have other cholesterol abnormalities, such as low HDL cholesterol or a high triglycerides level, you may be prescribed a drug combination or drugs and supplements.

Statins are generally safe drugs, but like all medications, they do have adverse side effects. Most are minor, such as stomach distress. However, liver damage can rarely occur. To make sure this doesn't happen, people who are put on statins need to undergo a blood test. Follow-up tests also may be ordered at the doctor's discretion, or if any other medication is added that may also cause liver problems.

Another rare side effect is rhabdomyolysis, a serious disease that causes muscle and kidney damage. Not uncommonly, people on statins experience muscle aches, which are usually not serious. But, if this happens, the doctor will order a CPK test, which measures the level of creatine phosphokinase in the blood. This enzyme is predominantly in muscle tissue. If the total CPK level is steeply elevated, this indicates that rhabdomyolysis may be occurring, and the statin will be stopped. The CPK test is not used when you begin taking a statin because some people do normally have elevated levels of this substance in their blood; however, some doctors do order this as a baseline test, especially when using two drugs together that have the risk of causing it.

Statins do not work for everyone, and because of their adverse side effects, some people cannot take them. Other types of medication that are used, either alone or in combination with a statin, are described below in alphabetical order.

Chapter Five

Bile acid sequestrants (known also as bile acid resins) bind with cholesterol-containing bile acids in the intestines and are then eliminated in the stool. These medications can produce smaller reductions in LDL cholesterol than can the statins (about 10–30 percent), but they also have the advantage of being extremely safe because they are excreted, not absorbed by the body. These drugs may produce a variety of symptoms, including constipation, bloating, nausea, and gas. Nowadays, these drugs are often used in combination with a statin if an additional cholesterol-reducing effect is needed. Examples of these drugs are Questran and Questran Light (cholestyramine), Colestid (colestipol), and WelChol (colesevelam).

Ezetimibe (Zetia) is the first in a new class of drugs that lower cholesterol in a new way. The drug lowers cholesterol by inhibiting its absorption through the wall of the intestine. Since only a small amount of the drug is absorbed into the body, it appears to be quite safe. This drug lowers the LDL cholesterol about 18 percent, which is not that much when you compare it to a statin. On the other hand, it can be valuable when used in combination with statins or for people who cannot take statins.

Fibrates are primarily effective in lowering triglycerides and, to a lesser extent, in increasing HDL cholesterol levels. Gemfibrozil (Lopid), the fibrate most widely used, and now available generically, is not that effective for lowering LDL cholesterol but is useful for people with high triglyceride levels. The reductions in triglycerides are generally 20–50 percent, with increases in HDL cholesterol of 10–15 percent. Another fibrate is fenofibrate, which is available under several brand names, including Tricor.

On the Road to Recovery

Nicotinic acid (Niacin) is a water-soluble B vitamin that you'll find in your daily vitamin supplement. But, to affect cholesterol, much higher dosages are prescribed. Although niacin is inexpensive and available without a prescription, it should not be used in these larger doses without a doctor's supervision because of potential side effects. Niacin reduces LDL cholesterol levels by 10–20 percent, reduces triglycerides by 20–50 percent, and raises HDL cholesterol by 15–35 percent. When it is used with simvastatin, one of the statins, the resulting rise in HDL can be dramatic. However, niacin is not that easy to tolerate; it can cause stomach discomfort, flushing, tingling, and headaches. In addition, it can increase blood glucose levels, so it is usually not used for people with diabetes. Examples of niacin are Nicolar and Niaspan. Nicotinamide, another form of the vitamin niacin, does not lower cholesterol levels and should not be used in its place.

Diuretics

Diuretic drugs, sometimes called "water pills," reduce the amount of salt and water in the body. They are used to help lower blood pressure, and although they were out of favor for a while, they are now highly recommended. These medications are also important when used to treat heart failure and for fluid retention. There are different classes of diuretic medicines. Each type works a little differently, but they all lower the amount of salt and water in the body, which helps to lower blood pressure. Some of the most popular diuretics are furosemide (Lasix) and bumetamide (Bumex). These are very powerful and may require a potassium supplement. Other, less powerful diuretics may not require such a supplement, especially if they are used in low dosage (such as hydrochlorthiazide) or in combination with a diuretic that causes potassium retention. Some medications combine two types of diuretics: one that tends to cause potassium loss and one that causes potassium retention. They include Dyazide, Aldactazide, and Maxzide. Another diuretic that helps retain potassium is spironolactone. Its first cousin, eplernone (Inspra), has been approved to treat high blood pressure and heart failure. These are just some diuretics; there are many more available.

Digitalis Medicines

Digitalis medicines strengthen the force of the heartbeat by binding with receptors in the cells of the heart that stop calcium from leaving them. As the calcium builds up, it causes the heartbeat to become stronger. Digitalis medicines are used to treat atrial fibrillation, an arrhythmia. Digitalis can improve the symptoms of congestive heart failure, and it used to be employed as the main treatment for it, but ACE inhibitors and beta blockers are now used instead because they also slow the disease's progression. Digitalis is only used in addition to these other medications to add to their effects.

STRAIGHT TALK ON MEDICATIONS

Taking medications correctly is very important. When you are taking multiple drugs, as most heart attack survivors do, and they have different dosing schedules, this can become downright tricky. Here are some tips:

- Learn how much of the medication you should take, how often you should take it, and whether or not it should be taken with food. Be consistent with your schedule and dosages. Use pill organizers or dispensers if you need help in remembering to take your pills.

- Take exact doses as prescribed by your doctor. Never intentionally skip or add doses.
- Consult your doctor before you stop taking a cardiovascular medication. Sometimes the effect of a drug may not be immediately apparent. This does not mean that the drug is not working.
- Over-the-counter nonsteroidal anti-inflammatory medications (like Aleve and Motrin) and aspirin may cause the body to retain sodium and water and may decrease the effect of an ACE inhibitor. NSAIDs may also interfere with the effect of aspirin. Check with your doctor before taking any anti-inflammatory medications.
- Keep your medicines in their original containers; don't mix them in the bottle with others.
- Take your medicine at the same time each day, at a time that is easy to remember, such as before meals, after work, or at bedtime.
- Do not take any over-the-counter (non-prescription) medications, such as aspirin, antacids, vitamins, or nutritional supplements, without consulting your doctor or pharmacist. Many of these can cause harmful interactions with others. Aspirin, for instance, can increase the risk of bleeding when taken with certain other over-the-counter medications.
- Store your medicines at room temperature, away from moisture, and out of direct sunlight. Don't store them in your refrigerator. Some medications lose their strength

Chapter Five

after a few months; if a medication is more than six months old, contact your doctor or pharmacist to determine if it should be discontinued or replaced.

- Plan ahead for a trip. Take twice as much medication with you as you expect to need. Pack half of your drugs in your luggage; carry on your person a second supply that could last several days. This way, if either your purse or luggage is lost or stolen, you still have an adequate supply for your trip.

- Make a written list of your medications, the times you take them, and the dosages, and carry it with you at all times.

- Remember, the drugs you take are intended for you alone, not for your spouse, neighbor, or friend. Likewise, you should never take another person's medication.

- Many cardiovascular drugs are very powerful and may have side effects, such as fatigue, depression, fainting, and dizziness. If you experience any such occurrence, contact your doctor.

SIX

Dealing with Complications

Thanks to advances in medical treatments, more and more women are surviving major heart attacks. But major heart attacks can result in serious heart damage—and the more serious the heart damage, the greater the chance of complications. Fortunately, the success in treating these complications is also increasing. The important thing to remember is that, if you do have complications, you need to understand what they are, and you need to work with your doctor to make sure they are properly treated.

The two main types of heart attack complications that occur after a heart attack are arrhythmias and congestive heart failure.

ARRHYTHMIAS (IRREGULAR HEARTBEATS)

An arrhythmia is the name given to any variation in the normal rhythm of the heart. Arrhythmias can be very minor, but they can also be serious. Sometimes very serious, even fatal, arrhythmias can occur immediately following a heart attack. This is why, after your heart attack, your heartbeat was carefully monitored while

Chapter Six

you were in the hospital. But an arrhythmia can appear weeks, months, or even years after the heart attack occurred. When this happens, the arrhythmia can seem to appear suddenly, seemingly out of the blue. But, upon testing, it may be discovered that the arrhythmia was caused by the damage that occurred from the heart attack.

How Arrhythmias Occur

An arrhythmia is caused by damage to your heart's electrical system. The beating of your heart is regulated by an electrical system located within the tissue of the heart muscle itself. This tissue contains a specialized group of cells, the sinus node, which has the ability to generate electrical energy on its own. These electrical impulses spread over the heart, causing the heart to contract about 100,000 times a day. The result is a normal heart rhythm of around 72 beats per minute.

It is perfectly normal for healthy people to experience irregularities in their heart rhythm. This is because all of the tissue in the heart—not only the sinus node—is capable of originating heartbeats. Sometimes this can occur harmlessly and is known as a premature atrial contraction (PAC) or premature ventricular contraction (PVC), depending on whether it occurs in the upper or lower chamber of the heart. Virtually everyone experiences these harmless heartbeats every day, although most of us remain unaware of them.

But damage to the heart's electrical system can result in more serious heartbeat irregularities. How much of a problem they are, though, depends on the type of damage and where in the heart it occurred. Arrhythmias are characterized according to where they occur in the heart. Those that occur in the upper chambers of the

Dealing with Complications

heart (the atria) are called atrial arrhythmias. Those that start in the lower chambers (the ventricles) are called ventricular arrhythmias. Generally, the arrhythmias that occur in the upper chambers of the heart are not as serious as those that occur in the lower chambers, especially after a heart attack.

An arrhythmia can be discovered in different ways. Your doctor may find it by listening to your heart. Or you may experience symptoms such as weakness, chest discomfort, shortness of breath, palpitations, dizziness, or fainting.

Upper Chamber Arrhythmias

Arrhythmias occur in either the upper or lower chambers of the heart. First we will look at upper chamber arrhythmias.

Atrial fibrillation: Also known as AF, this is the most common type of irregular heartbeat, affecting millions of women. Normally, the heart's electrical impulses originate in the sinus node in the atrium and travel in an orderly fashion from the upper chambers to the lower chambers of the heart. In AF, this orderly travel sequence is disrupted. Instead, the impulses originate chaotically throughout the atrium, bombarding the atrioventricular node in a disorganized fashion, before activating the ventricles. This results in a very rapid and irregular heartbeat that can go up to 300 beats per minute.

Normally, the impulses that originate in the upper portion of the heart cause the upper part to act in concert with the contractions that occur in the lower part. With AF, though, this synchronization is lost. The result can be a 30 percent loss in the heart's pumping efficiency. This can cause the heart to enlarge, or result in congestive heart failure, which is the other most common type of heart attack complication.

AF can result in symptoms such as heart palpitations, sweating, dizziness, and feeling faint. Other symptoms may include chest pain, pressure or discomfort, shortness of breath, or anxiety. Such symptoms can range from barely noticeable to frightening and disabling. Since these episodes also are unpredictable, they can cause great emotional distress.

Although usually not life threatening in itself, atrial fibrillation can cause serious problems. Women with AF have five times the risk of stroke because the irregular blood flow associated with AF can cause clots to form in the heart, and these can travel to the brain. Atrial fibrillation is diagnosed by using a monitoring device designed to detect arrhythmias. Treatment is aimed at slowing the rapid heart rate, and sometimes at restoring a regular heartbeat. Additional treatments may include medication, implantation of a pacemaker, or use of a technique known as radiofrequency ablation. A blood thinner (warfarin or Coumadin) may be prescribed to minimize the possibility of a stroke.

Atrial flutter: This condition is related to AF. Like AF, it causes a rapid, excessive heartbeat—150–300 beats per minute—but the atria beat in an organized manner, unlike the disorganized way that occurs with AF. Atrial flutter, though, can cause the same complications as atrial fibrillation, and it is diagnosed and treated in a similar way. One form of atrial flutter can actually be cured by radiofrequency ablation, but a much simpler version than that used to treat atrial fibrillation.

Sick sinus syndrome: This type of arrhythmia is a malfunction of the heart's primary natural pacemaker, the sinoatrial node that is located at the top of the right atrium. The scarring that results from a heart attack can cause sick sinus syndrome.

Dealing with Complications

This condition can cause palpitations, dizziness, fatigue, confusion, and chest pain.

Bradycardia, a type of sick sinus syndrome, is a too-slow heartbeat. Bradycardias are also classified into different types:

- *Inappropriate sinus bradycardia:* A condition in which the heart rate falls below 60 beats per minute and does not increase, even during exercise. This condition can cause fatigue and fainting.
- *Tachycardia-bradycardia syndrome:* A condition in which the heart alternates between beating too fast (tachycardia) and too slow (bradycardia).
- *Inappropriate sinus arrest:* A condition that occurs when the principal pacemaker cells in the sinus node fail to activate properly, causing a delay. If this persists, it can cause dizziness or lightheadedness.
- *Sinoatrial block*: A condition in which electrical impulses occur but do not travel to the rest of the heart.

Bradycardias can be treated in different ways. Sometimes they may be caused by medication, in which case an adjustment in the types of drugs used can eliminate the problem. If medication is not the cause, then the solution is often the implantation of a pacemaker.

Heart block: Another heart rhythm disorder is caused by an interruption in the passage of impulses through the heart's electrical system. The problem here is that the impulses, which start in the heart's upper chambers, do not reach the lower ones. There are three different degrees of heart block.

Chapter Six

First-degree heart block means the impulse is somewhat slowed but does not stop, no symptoms may occur, and it may not cause any problem. There are two types of second-degree heart block: Type I and Type II. Both types may have such short disruptions as to cause no symptoms, or they may appear as dizziness or even fainting. Type II is the more serious of these two types. In third-degree heart block, known also as complete heart block, the upper and lower heart chambers are completely separated electrically. This results in a slow heart rate that can cause fatigue, fainting, and congestive heart failure.

Heart block does not necessarily grow worse, but if it does, it can lead to a problem known as Stokes-Adams attacks, a condition that involves fainting and can sometimes cause convulsions as well. If fainting is occurring, a pacemaker can be implanted. In some cases, heart block may occur only temporarily after a heart attack. In this case, the need for a pacemaker may be temporary as well. Mild cases of heart block may require no treatment.

Lower Chamber Arrhythmias

Ventricular tachycardia: As noted earlier in this chapter, the heart's natural pacemaker is located in the sinus node; however, all of the heart's tissue is capable of generating heartbeats. In ventricular tachycardia, the scarring of the heart, which results from heart damage due to a heart attack, can leave pockets of heart tissue that begin acting like a pacemaker, sending out impulses. Ventricular tachycardia is a potentially fatal disruption of the heartbeat that may cause the heart to become unable to pump adequate blood through the body. The heart rate may be 100–300 beats per minute (normal is 60–100).

Dealing with Complications

The symptoms of ventricular tachycardia include low blood pressure, dizziness or lightheadedness, shortness of breath, and even loss of consciousness. This condition must be treated as a medical emergency. Although an extra beat or two of the heart is harmless, lots of extra beats can cause havoc, especially when they are weak and disorganized. Such fast, weak, and disorganized heartbeats cannot generate enough blood to flow throughout the body. The result can be a very serious, and even potentially fatal, heart condition.

Ventricular fibrillation (VF) is a severely abnormal heart rhythm that, unless treated immediately, causes death. VF is responsible for 75–85 percent of sudden deaths in people with heart problems. The main symptom of VF is that the person suddenly collapses or falls unconscious, because the brain and muscles have stopped receiving blood from the heart. If the person is not immediately resuscitated, sudden death can occur. Within one hour before the collapse (or sudden death from VF), some people complain of symptoms such as chest pain, palpitations, shortness of breath, dizziness, or nausea.

DIAGNOSING AND TREATING ARRHYTHMIAS

Obviously, given the seriousness of some arrhythmias, diagnosing the condition before an attack occurs is critically important. Arrhythmias are usually diagnosed with a series of heart monitor tests.

Ventricular arrhythmias can be treated with intravenous medication or by an electrical shock to the heart, which is known as electrical cardioversion or defibrillation. The implantation of an ICD is proving to be a lifesaver for people with these types of arrhythmias.

An automatic implantable cardioverter defibrillator (ICD), a device about the size of a small cell phone, is surgically implanted in the chest. It can quickly detect an abnormal heart rhythm and convert the arrhythmia back to normal rhythm by delivering an electrical shock to the heart. This way the ICD can effectively prevent sudden death.

An automated external defibrillator (AED) does the same thing. This is a portable device that is not implanted but is applied on the outside of the body. Putting AEDs in public places, such as offices, schools, and golf courses, or even in the home, is becoming more commonplace.

CONGESTIVE HEART FAILURE

Congestive heart failure, known also as simply "heart failure," sounds worse than it actually is. This term doesn't mean that the heart has actually *failed* but that it is now unable to adequately pump blood throughout the body because of damage from a heart attack. Early diagnosis and proper treatment are important to prevent this condition from becoming worse.

How Congestive Heart Failure Occurs

When your heart is damaged by a heart attack, it may undergo a natural process called "remodeling," in an attempt to compensate for the damage. If, for instance, the left ventricle (the main pumping station) is damaged, the heart must work harder. During this remodeling process, the heart's walls grow thicker, and the bottom part of the heart grows larger and more spherical. Although your heart is making these changes to keep up with its workload, ultimately they cause the heart to become weaker. This process is what gives this condition the name "heart failure," because the heart is becoming weaker, or *failing*.

Unfortunately, this failure to work properly also causes the heart's contractions to become weaker. Since not enough blood is reaching the body, the body begins increasing its own blood volume to make up for the shortfall. Because the weakened heart cannot provide enough blood to the kidneys, the body secretes a hormone known as aldosterone. This hormone prompts the body to retain water and sodium as a means of increasing volume. This results in a backing up of fluid within the body that results in shortness of breath and is why people with congestive heart failure are said to be "retaining water."

Congestive heart failure can occur in the left side or the right side of the heart, or both. The heart is composed of two pumps, which work in concert. The left side pumps oxygen-filled blood out to the rest of the body. Then this supply of oxygen-rich blood comes into the heart from the right side, which pumps the blood into the lungs. In left-sided heart failure, the left side of the heart isn't working properly. In right-sided heart failure, the right side of the heart is inadequately pumping. Since both sides of the pump depend on the other, if the right side of the heart isn't working correctly, the left side will not have enough blood to pump. If the left side of the heart works poorly, the problem "backs up" to the right side and results in inadequate function. As a result, the most common cause of right-sided heart failure is left-sided heart failure.

Congestive heart failure is historically classified into four groups, ranging from Class 1 to Class 4, depending on how much exertion is needed to bring on symptoms. It's important to remember, though, that sometimes the seeming severity of the symptoms do not match the degree of the heart's functional impairment. Someone with serious congestive heart failure may have no symptoms, while someone with a less impaired heart may seem to have worse symptoms. It isn't known why this is so, but it may have something to do with the way the body compensates for the loss in the heart's pumping function. A more recent classification of heart failure divides heart failure into stages A through D, depending on whether you have risk factors for heart failure, severe heart failure, or a problem with severity in between.

Although they can both occur at the same time, two distinctions are made between the types of heart failure: *diastolic heart failure* and *systolic heart failure*. About 50–60 percent of people develop systolic heart failure, in which the heart becomes weak. In diastolic heart failure, the heart pumps well, but the muscle has become too stiff. Diastolic heart failure occurs in about 40–50 percent of people who have heart failure. This condition is most commonly caused by high blood pressure.

DIAGNOSING AND TREATING CONGESTIVE HEART FAILURE

Currently, there are no treatments that can cure congestive heart failure, but the condition can be successfully managed. So, if you've had a heart attack, your doctor must determine if your heart function remains strong. If you've had anything but the mildest heart attack, a heart function test should be part of your follow-up cardiac examinations in the coming years. If your doctor suspects your heart's function might have been compromised, treatment should begin immediately. If you develop symptoms or clinical signs of congestive heart failure, it is very important that your doctor investigate further. This is particularly true if your heart attack was caused by coronary heart disease, in which the narrowed coronary arteries did not allow enough blood to get to the heart, resulting in the apparent death of some of the heart muscle tissue. This tissue may not actually have died; the sudden stoppage of blood may have just "stunned" it. In such a case, angioplasty or coronary artery bypass surgery can restore the blood flow, bringing this seemingly dead heart muscle to life.

The Symptoms of Congestive Heart Failure

The most common symptoms of heart failure are feeling very tired and being short of breath. Shortness of breath can occur with exertion or simply lying flat in bed. People with heart failure may wake up panting or gasping for breath, or may find that they have to sleep on more pillows to breathe comfortably in bed. In the early stages, they may cough; later on, they may bring up bloody or frothy sputum. Rapid weight gain or bodily swelling is caused by an accumulation of fluid in the body, which is usually noticed in the legs and ankles. These symptoms may not necessarily be present at the same time.

Initially, the most important treatment for heart failure is done to alleviate symptoms. At the same time, it's very important to discover what caused the condition. In some cases, the cause of heart failure can be reversed if blood flow is restored to the heart. Coronary bypass surgery or balloon angioplasty can be used if the cause of heart failure is the diminished blood flow to the heart caused by coronary heart disease. A damaged heart valve that is causing the heart to overwork can also be surgically replaced or repaired.

But, often, the cause of the heart failure is not reversible. Then, the goal of treatment becomes strengthening the heart, managing symptoms, and slowing the progression of the disease.

Treating Congestive Heart Failure

The treatment of heart failure has changed somewhat over the past several years. Treatment now begins earlier and more aggressively, ideally before symptoms occur or as soon as possible thereafter. Other changes have occurred as well. Years ago, if you had congestive heart failure, you were told to rest; today, you're given an exercise program. Although exercise does not strengthen the heart muscle itself, regular physical activity enables the cardiovascular system to work more efficiently and effectively, so you can do more. Salt restriction and controlling high blood pressure are very important. Medication is also used. Pacing devices are sometimes needed or, as a last resort, cardiac transplantation.

Medication

Most of the time, congestive heart failure is treated with medication. In fact, people with this condition generally take several medications daily. These drugs are very important; different ones work in different ways, and they are often used in different combinations to best manage heart failure. Here's a rundown on the ones most commonly used to treat congestive heart failure. For more details, see the previous chapter on drugs.

- *ACE inhibitors:* Now an important part of treating systolic heart failure, these drugs not only improve heart failure symptoms but slow the progressive nature of the disease as well.

- *Angiotensin II receptor blockers:* This newer class of drugs has an effect similar to that of ACE inhibitors but causes fewer side effects in some people.
- *Beta blockers:* Beta blockers are now considered an effective treatment for heart failure, but they used to be considered harmful, because they blunt the effects of adrenaline, the hormone in the body that makes the heart beat fast and hard, which was considered desirable in heart failure patients. Newer studies have found that beta blockers stabilize heart rhythm, improve the heart's functioning, prevent further weakening of heart muscle, prevent additional heart attacks, and prolong life.
- *Digitalis:* Extracted from the foxglove plant, digitalis is one of the oldest cardiac drugs. The drug causes the heart to beat more forcefully, improves circulation, and prevents recurrent heart failure. Digitalis does not, however, slow the progression of congestive heart failure or prolong life.
- *Spironolactone:* This hormone, produced by the kidneys, is sometimes prescribed for patients with severe congestive heart failure to improve symptoms and prolong longevity. A synthetic version of this hormone is also available.
- *Diuretics:* Diuretics help the kidneys rid the body of excess water and sodium, reducing swelling throughout the body and congestion in the lungs.

Pacing Devices

Regular pacemakers, the kind used to treat slow heartbeats, are not used to treat congestive heart failure, but there are specialized pac-

Chapter Six

ing devices that can help. One is a device that performs an action known as "biventricular pacing." This involves implanting three wires into the heart that can be used to stimulate different parts of the heart to contract in a more efficient manner. This can enable patients with heart failure to feel better when the other treatments they are using are not working as well as they should be.

Also, some women with congestive heart failure due to a heart attack, or those with moderately or severely weakened heart muscles, may live longer if they have a defibrillator implanted. This small, surgically implanted device monitors the heart rate and sends an electric signal to restore a too-rapid heart rhythm back to normal.

Cardiac Transplantation

For patients with severely damaged hearts, heart transplantation may be the only alternative. Waiting for a donor heart can be a lengthy process, so sometimes a left ventricular assist device (LVAD) is used to aid the heart in the meantime, as a bridge to transplantation. The LVAD is a mechanically powered pump that is implanted in the abdomen and assists the heart until a transplant can be performed. The LVAD may also be used as a more permanent device for people who are not considered candidates for cardiac transplantation.

Developing complications as the result of a heart attack can seem daunting, but the important thing to remember it that there are now many effective ways to diagnose and treat these problems. The goal is to manage these complications so that you can lead a long, healthy life.

SEVEN

Managing High Blood Pressure

Uncontrolled high blood pressure significantly raises your risk of having another heart attack or developing congestive heart failure, kidney disease, or stroke. Controlling it is not easy, but it is essential. And the payoff is big: by controlling your high blood pressure, you can significantly reduce your heart attack risk.

Blood pressure is the force of blood against artery walls. It rises and falls during the day. When it stays elevated over time, the condition is known as high blood pressure, or hypertension.

HOW HIGH BLOOD PRESSURE
DAMAGES YOUR HEART

Blood pressure provides a measurement of how hard your heart needs to work in order to pump blood through the body. The higher your blood pressure, the more resistance there is to the flowing blood, so the harder your heart must pump. Obviously, you want your heart to work less, not more, so it's important to lower this resistance by lowering your blood pressure.

Chapter Seven

If your blood pressure is too high, this can damage your heart in two important ways. High blood pressure contributes to atherosclerosis, which is the buildup of fatty deposits within your arteries that narrows them, setting the stage for another heart attack.

High blood pressure also can result in a form of heart disease called "hypertensive cardiovascular disease," which causes your heart to become thickened, enlarged, and eventually weakened.

Just a small rise in blood pressure can cause serious health problems. For most people, a relatively small rise in blood pressure can translate to a doubling of the risk of heart attack, congestive heart failure, stroke, or kidney disease.

WHAT CAUSES HIGH BLOOD PRESSURE?

Blood pressure increases as people age, particularly after they reach 60, and blood vessels become stiffer. But not everyone over 60 develops high blood pressure, and this certainly doesn't explain the development of high blood pressure in people who are much younger. This is why the vast majority of high blood pressure cases—about 94 percent—are said to occur for no discernible reason. This type of high blood pressure is called "essential hypertension." The remaining 6 percent of people with high blood pressure develop it due to an underlying condition. This is "secondary hypertension," or "identifiable hypertension," which means that the high blood pressure is caused by a disease or condition that is correctable. This happens so infrequently, though, that unless there is some obvious evidence that you have such a problem (you've been diagnosed with Cushing's syndrome, for instance), your doctor generally will not look for such an ailment, assume you have essential hypertension, and treat it. If your blood pressure

Managing High Blood Pressure

cannot be controlled with medication, then your doctor may investigate further to determine if you have one of these underlying causes of high blood pressure.

These are the causes of correctable hypertension:

- Sleep apnea, which occurs in people whose breathing stops frequently while they are asleep.
- Primary aldosteronism, which is a rare disorder of the adrenal glands.
- Renovascular disease, a rare disease of the blood vessels of the kidneys.
- Chronic kidney disease.
- Thyroid disease.
- Cushing's syndrome, a rare disorder in which the body produces too much of the hormone cortisol.
- Coarctation of the aorta, a congenital defect in which a portion of the aorta is narrowed or pinched, which reduces blood flow to the heart.
- Pheochromocytoma, a rare tumor usually in the adrenal glands.

There are also certain habits, drugs, and foods that can contribute to high blood pressure. Oral contraceptives can raise blood pressure, although this effect often goes away after the medication is discontinued. Certain other drugs can also cause high blood pressure, including:

- Nonsteroidal anti-inflammatory drugs (NSAIDS), including aspirin and ibuprofen
- Steroids

Chapter Seven

- Decongestants
- Cocaine, amphetamines, and other illicit drugs
- Over-the-counter diet supplements, including ephedra, ma haung, bitter orange
- Also, while it's not a drug, black licorice can raise blood pressure

Cigarette smoking contributes to high blood pressure because nicotine causes blood vessels to constrict and makes the heart beat faster. People who habitually drink too much alcohol can also develop high blood pressure, and this can also make blood pressure more difficult to control. People with diabetes and those who are obese are also more likely to develop high blood pressure.

A diet too high in salt has also been linked to the development of high blood pressure. Being under stress is another contributor.

BLOOD PRESSURE CLASSIFICATION

Blood pressure is measured in millimeters of mercury (mmHg) and recorded as two numbers—systolic pressure (as the heart beats and pumps blood) over diastolic pressure (as the heart relaxes between beats). Both numbers are important.

Over the years, it's been found that high blood pressure poses more risk than thought previously, so the classifications have become increasingly stringent. Many people whose blood pressure readings previously were considered within a normal range are now classified as having "prehypertension." This means that although they don't have high blood pressure now, they are likely to develop it. In fact, we now know that those with normal blood pressure at age 55–65 have a 90 percent chance of developing high blood pressure over the next 20 years.

The blood pressure classifications are as follows:

- *Normal:* Less than 120 systolic and less than 80 diastolic.
- *Prehypertension:* 120–139 systolic or 80–89 diastolic.
- *Stage 1 hypertension:* 140–159 systolic or 90–99 diastolic.
- *Stage 2 hypertension:* 160 or more systolic and 100 or more diastolic.
- *White-coat hypertension:* This is not a part of the official classification system, but it is an important category, because it denotes people who experience a temporary rise in blood pressure when they become anxious as their doctor takes their blood pressure. Blood pressure monitoring at home or with ambulatory electronic monitors can distinguish white-coat hypertension from the real thing.
- *Masked or reverse white-coat hypertension:* This refers to blood pressure that is normal in the doctor's office but elevated elsewhere. This form of high blood pressure is a more recently recognized category of hypertension.

If your blood pressure is high enough to reach Stage 1, you have high blood pressure. There is no such thing as "mild" high blood pressure. Any blood pressure reading above "normal" needs to be taken seriously, although the aggressiveness of the type of treatment varies depending on how high the blood pressure is and what associated risk factors or vascular disease may also be present.

Chapter Seven

Bear in mind also that risk does not increase according to a simple rise in blood pressure; once you get into the higher numbers, such as Stage 2, your risk more rapidly escalates, putting you in extreme danger, over time, of a heart attack or stroke.

DIAGNOSING HIGH BLOOD PRESSURE

High blood pressure is known as the "silent killer" for the simple reason that blood pressure can climb quite high—even into the danger zone—without your even realizing that something is amiss. People with high blood pressure can occasionally experience headaches, nosebleeds, and shortness of breath, but this is the exception; the vast majority of people with high blood pressure do not experience any symptoms. Heart attack survivors may only learn they have high blood pressure at the time of their heart attack.

This is why the practice of having your blood pressure taken is such a common part of a doctor's appointment. It is so common that you're unlikely to question how it's done. But sometimes medical professionals (doctors, nurses, nurse practitioners, and physician's assistants) don't follow the proper procedure and may get an inaccurate blood pressure reading as a result. Make sure that your blood pressure is taken properly. Rather than having your blood pressure taken while you sit on an examination table with your legs dangling, you should be seated quietly for at least five minutes before the procedure begins.

It is also important that your blood pressure be taken with the right-sized cuff for the width of your upper arm. If the cuff is too small, you may appear to have high blood pressure, even if you do not. This usually occurs more often with men than women but can happen to a woman if she has a wide upper arm. Also, your doctor should tell you your specific blood pressure measurements and your blood pressure goals, so you can see what you need to aim for. Get this in writing, so you can refer to it.

It's estimated that 60 percent of diabetics have high blood pressure. If you fall into this category, the need for you to control your blood pressure becomes even more urgent, because having both diabetes and high blood pressure raises the risk of another heart attack even more steeply. But, too often, diabetes treatment focuses solely on blood glucose control, which may be why diabetics are so likely to have another heart attack, develop congestive heart failure, or suffer a stroke. So, it's important to make sure that your doctor pays attention to your blood pressure as well.

Congestive heart failure can result from the combination of coronary heart disease and high blood pressure. As a heart attack survivor, you're at risk for developing this complication, so this is another reason to control your blood pressure.

SUCCESSFULLY MANAGING HIGH BLOOD PRESSURE

Managing high blood pressure is not easy. If you have a high level of LDL cholesterol, the "bad" cholesterol, for instance, it's very likely that you can lower it to a normal level by using one of the statin drugs. Although high blood pressure drugs are effective, they don't work as effectively for everyone with high blood pressure as the statins do for LDL cholesterol. This is why, after decades of public education and the development of numerous medications, only one-third of the people with high blood pressure succeed in controlling their blood pressure. But this is not going to happen in your case, because you and your doctor are going to work together to make sure you reach this important goal.

Monitoring Blood Pressure at Home

Most people find that monitoring their blood pressure at home is a useful way to make sure that their blood pressure medication is working, and to provide extra motivation to stay on their blood pressure lowering regimen. These units can be found at almost any discount store or pharmacy, or they can be ordered easily online.

There are two different main styles of home blood pressure monitoring units: the traditional type that uses a cuff and a pump, and an electronic type that gives the digital reading automatically and may be easier to use. No matter which type you use, make sure the cuff fits properly around your upper arm. If you do have a wide upper arm, purchase a larger cuff, which is usually sold separately.

High Blood Pressure Medication

Usually at least two and sometimes three or four different drugs are required for successful blood pressure control. These drugs may need to be taken at different times. Also, many people tend to associate high blood pressure medications with adverse side effects—whether this is warranted or not. Nowadays, though, there are some seven different classes of blood pressure medications, and multiple drugs within each class, so eventually your doctor should be able to find the right combination to control your blood pressure with few, if any, side effects. But this means you need to notify your doctor of any side effects you may experience, and patiently go through a trial-and-error procedure to find just the right combination.

By taking this approach, you should be able to master your drug regimen and find the combination that will control your high blood pressure with a minimum of side effects. But, if your blood pressure remains high and your doctor has exhausted the attempts to lower it, ask for a referral to a blood pressure specialist. Lowering your blood pressure risk is worth it. For more about medication, see the previous chapter.

Lifestyle Changes to Manage High Blood Pressure

If you have normal blood pressure or fall into the "prehypertensive" category, eating healthily and exercising may prevent you from developing high blood pressure. If you have high blood pressure, these measures may help you lower it, but you'll probably need medication as well. However, watching your diet and being active may enable you to reduce the amount of medication you need. Here are the lifestyle steps you need to take.

- *Lose weight, if you need to:* If you're overweight, losing weight should lower your blood pressure. In fact, loss of some 20 pounds can result in a reduction of 5–20 mmHg in your systolic blood pressure. There are, however, a few things to bear in mind. First, not everyone is "weight responsive," which means that not every woman who loses weight will see the result translated in her blood pressure reading. If you follow a low-carbohydrate diet, you'll lose a lot of "water weight," at least initially, which may result in lower blood pressure. But, as your body becomes accustomed to your diet, this effect can wear off, and your blood pressure may rise again. Generally, though, following a sound weight-loss plan can result in a permanent lowering of blood pressure for most people.

- *Follow a healthy diet:* Healthy eating can help lower blood pressure. The DASH diet is a good way to do this. The DASH diet (the acronym stands for Dietary Approaches to Stop Hypertension) is clinically proved to lower high blood pressure, as well as high cholesterol and homocysteine, the amino acid in the blood that appears to increase the risk of heart disease. The DASH eating plan includes whole grains, poultry, fish, and nuts, and it has reduced amounts of fats, red meats, sweets, and sugared beverages. It is also rich in potassium, calcium, magnesium, fiber, and protein. The diet is distributed by the federal government through the National Heart, Lung, and Blood Institute, and you can download everything you need to follow it for free—including recipes—from www.nhlbi.nih.gov/health/public/heart/hbp/dash/ or by calling 301-592-8573.

- *Eat less salt:* The less salt you eat, the lower your blood pressure will be. It's as simple as that. Not everyone is sensitive to the effects of dietary salt, but if you have high blood pressure, it's more likely that you are. People with high blood pressure often think that if they avoid salt for a few weeks, their blood pressure will drop. This isn't so—it can take months to detect a possible difference. So stick with it. You should consume no more than 2,400 mg of salt daily, but it's estimated that Americans consume about 3,300 mg of salt a day in their foods. That figure may actually be about 4,000 mg if you add in the use of

Managing High Blood Pressure

the saltshaker. Here are some suggestions on how to cut down on salt:

—Banish your saltshaker from the table. If this is too difficult at first, gradually cut down the amount of salt you use. Use spices instead of salt at the table. Lemon, lime, vinegar, and salt-free seasoning blends are very tasty. If you want to use a salt substitute, check with your doctor first. Salt substitutes are high in potassium, and this can cause your potassium level to be too high if you have kidney disease or are on certain types of prescription medication. A too-high potassium level can cause a heartbeat irregularity.

—Buy reduced sodium or no-salt-added products.

—Buy fresh or plain frozen vegetables, instead of those that are canned with salt.

—Use fresh poultry, fish, and meat, rather than canned, smoked, or processed types.

—Avoid cured foods (such as bacon and ham) and pickled foods (including pickled vegetables, olives, and sauerkraut).

—Avoid such condiments as MSG, mustard, horseradish, catsup, and barbecue salt. If you use soy sauce or teriyaki sauce, choose low-sodium versions.

—When you cook, use fresh herbs or herb-flavored oils to flavor foods.

—Cook rice, pasta, and hot cereals without salt, even if the directions call for it.

—Choose salt-free or low-salt versions of convenience foods, such as pizza, canned soups or broths, and salad dressings.

—Buy tuna packed in water, or rinse it to get rid of some of the salt.

—When eating out, don't be shy. Talk to your waiter ahead of time and find out how the food is prepared. Choose dishes that can be prepared without salt. Most likely, the chef has received such requests before, and will be happy to accommodate you.

■ *Exercise regularly:* The regular exercise you'll be doing to reduce your heart attack risk should help control your blood pressure as well. This means doing aerobic exercise, such as brisk walking, jogging, swimming, or cycling for at least 30 minutes about five to seven days a week. Even if you cannot do that amount, just exercising one to one and a half hours a week has been found to help lower blood pressure.

Achieving your blood pressure goal is sometimes not easy; it can take a combination of medications along with lifestyle changes. But it is among the most worthwhile changes you can make, and it will help you prevent another heart attack.

EIGHT

Controlling Diabetes

THE DANGERS OF DIABETES

If you have diabetes, you are at greatly increased risk for suffering another heart attack. Therefore, you need to do all you can to prevent this from happening.

First, you need to learn to control your blood glucose (sugar) level.

Second, you must reduce all of the other risk factors you have that contributed to your heart attack.

Third, you must find an excellent doctor to work with, one who takes a proactive stand to make sure that, should your heart disease worsen, it will be promptly diagnosed and treated.

All of these steps are necessary because diabetes is such a serious risk factor. If you have diabetes, you are as likely as a non-diabetic heart attack survivor to suffer another heart attack, develop congestive heart failure, or die of a heart-related cause. So, you need to get your blood sugar level under control and keep it under control.

Chapter Eight

WHAT IS DIABETES?

Diabetes mellitus (the medical name for the most common form of diabetes) is a metabolic disorder in which the body's ability to metabolize glucose-using insulin, an important hormone, is impaired.

Diabetes usually indirectly accounts for many fatal illnesses. The formal cause of death may be listed as heart attack, heart failure, kidney disease, or stroke, but for many of its victims, the precursor was diabetes. Diabetes also accounts for a number of non-fatal but serious health problems, including blindness and amputations that result from poor circulation.

Diabetes causes all these complications—including setting the stage for a heart attack—because it damages virtually every vessel in the body, including the coronary arteries. Diabetes results in an excess amount of glucose in the blood; this blood becomes "glycosylated," which means that sugar attaches itself to the protein, an important component of blood. This makes the protein in the blood behave differently, and this unfavorably affects the blood vessels, leading to the formation and progression of plaque in the arteries. This results in coronary heart disease—as well as the tendency for the vessels themselves to lose their flexibility and become stiff. Diabetes also causes the blood to become more likely to clot, which increases heart attack risk.

As if that was not bad enough, diabetes also results in a low-level chronic inflammatory condition in your body. This is such a low level of inflammation that you are unaware of it, but this condition is now a leading suspect in the hunt for a cause of what sets off the process that results in coronary heart disease. So diabetes may not only create the conditions for atherosclerosis, but it may kick off the process itself.

Controlling Diabetes

"I had my heart attack when I was 58," Carol says. "It seemed to come out of the blue. I had gone to pick up my new car from the dealership that morning and, suddenly, I felt nauseous, sweaty, and lightheaded. I passed out, and when I came to, I was in the hospital. I was told I'd had a heart attack. Not only that, but that I was diabetic. That was a lot to contend with."

Carol is not unusual. Diabetes commonly develops an average of seven years before it's diagnosed, so it has a head start on causing damage. Therefore, it's not uncommon for women heart attack survivors to suddenly learn that they have two serious health threats to deal with, not just one.

Remember, though, there are steps you can take to reduce the risk of another heart attack. But it takes real motivation and a lot of work. You *must* make certain you receive the best medical care. You *must* follow your doctor's recommendations to the letter. You *must* do everything you can to lower *all* your heart attack risk factors. These are steps that all female heart attack survivors must do—but when you are diabetic, you really have *absolutely* no time to waste.

THE TYPES OF DIABETES

If you were recently diagnosed with diabetes, or developed it as an adult, you probably have Type II diabetes (formerly known as "adult-onset diabetes"), which is the most common form of the disease and accounts for about 90 percent of the cases. In this form of the disease, the body produces plenty of insulin but cannot use it properly. This type of diabetes used to develop almost exclusively in people over 40, but it is now being seen at higher rates in younger people, probably due to the growing rates of obesity and lack of exercise, as well as the increasing popularity of starchy and sugary foods. This type of diabetes is usually controlled with a combination of diet, exercise, and increasingly, oral medication. Some oral diabetes medications may do double duty, lowering heart attack risk as well. This is an ever changing field, with much research currently going on.

Usually, people with this form of diabetes do not need to take insulin, or if they do, it is only after they've had the disease for many years. But sometimes, after a heart attack, you may need to do so. This is because the biological stress on the body caused by the heart attack results in this need, either temporarily or indefinitely. It's also been found that diabetics who are put on insulin prior to coronary artery bypass surgery have better results. But this may only need to be a temporary measure, and you may eventually be able to stop taking insulin.

There are two other forms of diabetes. *Type I diabetes* (formerly called "juvenile diabetes") affects only about 10 percent of all diabetics. In this form of the disease, the body's ability to produce insulin is destroyed, so people with this form of diabetes must take insulin. *Gestational diabetes* occurs during pregnancy. Not every woman who develops gestational diabetes becomes diabetic later on, although the risk that this will occur is higher.

IMPAIRED GLUCOSE TOLERANCE (PRE-DIABETES)

Your doctor may have told you that you don't have diabetes but that you do have "pre-diabetes," or "impaired glucose tolerance" or "impaired fasting glucose." If this is the case, you must consider this condition as a very serious risk factor for another heart attack—as serious as if you'd been told you have diabetes.

Pre-diabetes is an increasingly common condition in which blood glucose levels are higher than normal but not yet diabetic. The medical term for this condition is "impaired glucose tolerance" or "impaired fasting glucose." But, no matter what the term used, the important fact is this—you are at increased risk of developing a full-fledged case of diabetes. The good news, however, is that you have bought some more time to make the lifestyle changes you must make in order to prevent it. So here are the three things you must do:

First, if you are overweight, you must lose that excess weight. By losing weight and exercising at least two and a half hours each week, you can greatly reduce the probability that you will develop diabetes. And you don't even need to lose that much weight—a slow weight loss of 1–2 pounds a week, amounting to a loss of 7–10 percent of your body weight, will help prevent the development of diabetes.

Second, you must begin a program of regular exercise.

Third, you must make sure your doctor monitors you, to ensure that your blood sugar levels improve, and that you do not develop diabetes.

MEETING YOUR DIABETES GOALS

After you have a heart attack, it may seem overwhelming to do all the things you must now do to stay in good health. But, as a diabetic, it remains extremely important that you also focus on the

Chapter Eight

goal of maintaining a favorable blood glucose level. By doing this, you may prevent the development—or slow the progression of—the complications of diabetes that affect the eyes, kidneys, and nerves. But you must also do this to reduce your risk of another heart attack.

Monitoring Your Glucose Level

There needs to be a certain amount of glucose, or sugar, in your blood to be metabolized into energy. This glucose level fluctuates throughout the day, depending on what you eat and your level of activity, among other factors. Diabetics must check their glucose levels several times a day to make sure that they are within a healthy range. So, work with your doctor or diabetes educator to learn what your ideal glucose levels are, when they should be checked, and how to use a glucose monitor.

You need to know what your ideal fasting blood glucose level is, as well as what it should be throughout the day. Your blood glucose levels should fall within the lower, normal, or intermediate range of these numbers—the lower the better. If your level is in the higher range, you are more likely to develop complications, and to develop them sooner.

In addition to your taking daily sugar level readings, your doctor takes a reading once every three months from a blood sample. This is known as the "Hb A_{Ic} level," which refers to the amount of glucose that coats the protein in your blood due to diabetes. This is also known as "glycosylated hemoglobin," or GHb. You should also know what this level should be, what your level is, and if it is not at goal, what steps your doctor says you need to take to reach it.

Controlling Diabetes

Choosing a Doctor

Because diabetes is a complicated disease, choosing a doctor who can help you keep it under control is very important. If your internist or primary care physician can successfully treat you, that's great. If your condition is difficult to control, ask your doctor for a referral to an endocrinologist. Endocrinologists are doctors who specialize in the treatment of metabolic and glandular disorders, including diabetes.

Your doctor also must be aware of the complications that diabetes can have on heart health. Heart disease is a progressive disease, and as a diabetic, you cannot rely on symptoms to tip you off that your heart disease is worsening, or that you may be on the brink of a heart attack. Diabetes can effectively mask the symptoms of a heart attack. This may be because neuropathy, a nerve disorder common in diabetics, can impair your body's ability to perceive sensation. As a result, some diabetics may not perceive the chest pain that may warn of an impending heart attack. In addition, a diabetic woman is more likely to suffer a "silent" heart attack, which is a heart attack that can be detected with tests, but of which the woman may be unaware because she experienced no symptoms at the time. This type of heart attack also causes heart damage.

Be sure to ask your doctor how he or she intends to monitor the health of your cardiovascular system. Currently, there are no specific guidelines that govern how often a diabetic who is not experiencing symptoms should undergo cardiac testing, but you should ask your doctor about it. The manner in which your doctor discusses this should tip you off to whether the issue of your diabetes is taken seriously.

Chapter Eight

Medication to Control Diabetes

As a heart attack survivor, you are probably already on several different kinds of medication. Being a diabetic increases the number of medications you will probably need to take. But medication is a tricky subject, and like everything else, diabetes makes it more complicated.

Some types of diabetes medications can improve your heart problems; on the other hand, some types of heart medication can lead to problems if you have diabetes. For instance, if you have diabetes, high blood pressure, and kidney disease, an ACE inhibitor or angiotension receptor blocker (ARB) is usually the drug of choice, because it benefits the heart, helps bring down blood pressure, and protects the kidneys. However, amlodipine (Norvasc), the most popular blood pressure medication, can potentially worsen kidney disease when used alone. Also, if you have diabetes, you should be taking an ACE inhibitor, because this type of drug reduces the risk of such deadly problems as heart attack and stroke. It may also prevent other complications of diabetes as well. If you have pre-diabetes or diabetes, you should consider taking a statin cholesterol-lowering drug, since that may reduce your heart attack risk.

NINE

Balancing Your Cholesterol Levels

Before you had your heart attack, your cholesterol levels may have been something you were aware of, but not necessarily concerned about. That's now changed following your heart attack. To prevent another heart attack, you now need not only to be concerned about your cholesterol levels—you need to improve them. That may be the case even if your cholesterol levels fall within the "normal" range. By keeping your cholesterol levels at goal, you can help reduce your heart attack risk. Fortunately, now more than ever, there is a lot you can do to accomplish this.

Start by discussing your current cholesterol levels with your doctor, and get your cholesterol levels—and your goal levels—in writing, so you can refer to them. Map out a strategy with your doctor to reach those goals. It will probably include diet and exercise, and depending on your current cholesterol levels, it may include cholesterol-lowering medication. But remember, there are lots of steps you can take to reach your cholesterol goals, and enjoying a glass of wine along with a handful of nuts may very well be included.

Chapter Nine

WHAT CHOLESTEROL IS
AND WHY IT IS IMPORTANT

Cholesterol, a component of your blood, is a soft, waxy, fat-like compound that belongs to a class of molecules called "sterols." Your liver manufactures about 85 percent of the cholesterol in your body; you absorb the additional 15 percent from the food you eat.

You need some amount of cholesterol in your body to survive. Cholesterol is found in cell membranes. It is used in the formation of the bile salts that help digest your food, and in the formation of your sex hormones. But an excessive amount of the cholesterol in your blood, especially certain types of it, increases heart attack risk.

Decades ago, when cholesterol first came to light as a dangerous risk factor, it was our total cholesterol number that mattered. Now, though, we know that our total cholesterol number is composed of different types of cholesterol, or fractions, and it is the different pattern that these components make that can contribute to that next heart attack.

THE THREE TYPES OF CHOLESTEROL

Basically, there are three kinds of cholesterol you need to know about: HDL cholesterol, LDL cholesterol, and triglycerides.

HDL cholesterol, or "high-density lipoprotein" cholesterol, is the "good" cholesterol. Your body manufactures this type of cholesterol for your protection; it removes excess cholesterol from the blood and transports it to the liver to be disposed. Its role in keeping your coronary arteries clear of blockages is commonly likened to how drain cleaner can keep the drains in your home clear.

Balancing Your Cholesterol Levels

Although all the cholesterol levels are important, it is HDL cholesterol which is the strongest cholesterol predictor of whether you will—or won't—have a heart attack, no matter what the rest of your cholesterol profile looks like. So remember, when it comes to HDL, high is good, and low is bad.

But, although most women who have heart attacks have HDL readings below the level considered desirable, it's impossible to generalize. Although it is less common, it is possible for you to have a heart attack, even if you have a high HDL cholesterol level. This is especially true if you have other risk factors, like smoking, a family history of heart disease, or diabetes.

But when it comes to HDL cholesterol, your goal is increasing this level—the higher the better. Since the concern about cholesterol came to light, the focus has been on LDL cholesterol, which is discussed next. This is because we have effective tools—mainly drugs—that can fight this form of cholesterol; finding strategies to raise HDL cholesterol has proven more elusive.

Also, although the recommendation for a desirable HDL level works for most people, it does not apply to some people—those who have an extremely low level of LDL cholesterol. This isn't common, but it does occur. In this case, having a high HDL level may not be that important, because there is much less LDL cholesterol for the HDL cholesterol to eliminate. So, in this case, a low HDL level may be acceptable.

LDL cholesterol, or "low-density lipoprotein" cholesterol, is the "bad" cholesterol. This type of cholesterol is deposited in the arterial wall, can form fatty streaks, and can help set the stage for another heart attack. So, when it comes to LDL cholesterol, the rule is: the lower the better.

Chapter Nine

Triglycerides, fatty compounds found in combination with LDL and low HDL cholesterol, are increasingly being seen as an important cause of heart disease. Triglycerides are the form of cholesterol in which your body stores and transports fat. Triglycerides alone increase heart disease risk, but not as significantly as do high LDL cholesterol or low HDL cholesterol. There is a see-saw relationship between triglycerides and HDL; generally, the higher the triglyceride level, the lower the HDL.

It's not unusual to have a heart attack even with a normal cholesterol level, so researchers are investigating the implications of breaking categories down into smaller patterns. These patterns involve different types of cholesterol fractions.

Because cholesterol and other fats can't dissolve in the blood, special carriers made of proteins called apoproteins transport them to and from the cells. When these apoproteins are joined with cholesterol and other substances, including triglycerides and phospholipids, they form compounds called lipoproteins. The density of these lipoproteins (and hence, the healthiness or un-healthiness of the cholesterol), is determined by the amount of each component in the lipoprotein molecule.

Although it was initially assumed that all LDL cholesterol patterns are harmful, some are more dangerous than are others. Currently, there are no generally agreed upon recommendations on when more precise testing should be done, but it may someday be useful. For instance, the statin-type drugs, which have become the cholesterol-lowering drug of choice, are less effective against the Lp(a) type of protein-cholesterol particle, which is related to LDL cholesterol. Lp(a) cholesterol is particularly harmful. Statin drugs, while effective against LDL cholesterol, are not very effective at lowering Lp(a), but niacin drugs are. This is the type of information that may someday be used to create a more personalized cholesterol-lowering regimen.

WHAT DETERMINES YOUR CHOLESTEROL BALANCE?

Your cholesterol level is determined by several factors. The most important factor is heredity, but other factors include age, diet, gender, obesity, other medical conditions, and smoking.

All people inherit the tendency to have high, normal, or low cholesterol levels. There are different types of inherited high cholesterol disorders. The most serious type is *familial homozygous.* This is a relatively rare condition in which both parents have inherited high cholesterol levels and they pass these genes on to their children. Only one in 1 million people inherit this condition, which results in alarmingly high total cholesterol levels. As a result, these people can develop heart disease in their teens or 20s. This condition is not affected by diet, so no matter what you eat, your cholesterol level will remain high.

Familial hyperlipidemia is a more common inherited high cholesterol condition that causes higher triglyceride levels and lower HDL levels, but it is affected by diet, so eating a healthy diet can improve it. There are inherited conditions that can also result in low HDL levels; some rare conditions can result in dramatically low ones.

Age also plays a large role. Generally, cholesterol levels tend to rise as we grow older, although cholesterol may level off, and even decrease, in the elderly. (It isn't known, though, if this appears to be the case because people with high LDL levels die earlier.) Gender also plays a role in cholesterol production. Prior to menopause, women generally have more favorable cholesterol levels than do men. After menopause, their cholesterol levels become less favorable, which is probably one reason why the risk of heart attacks in women begins to rise at this time. People with diabetes, both men and women, also tend to have unhealthy cholesterol profiles, the main problem being high triglycerides and low HDL's rather than very high LDL levels.

Being overweight generally translates into unhealthy cholesterol levels. This is especially true for women whose excess weight is located in their abdomen, as opposed to those who have heavier thighs and buttocks, which is why women who are "apple" shaped are believed to be more at risk for heart disease than their "pear" shaped counterparts.

The foods you eat contribute to your cholesterol levels. Those containing high levels of cholesterol, such as eggs, lean red meat, lobster, and shrimp, do not result in the high blood cholesterol levels if consumed in reasonably small quantities. However, foods high in saturated fats (even if these fats themselves do not contain cholesterol) can adversely affect your cholesterol levels. These include foods such as avocados, whole-milk dairy products, and well-marbled steaks. But adding to the confusion is that some people can eat foods high in cholesterol and saturated fats and yet have low cholesterol levels, whereas for others, the opposite is true—some people can follow a low-cholesterol diet and have high levels of cholesterol. This is probably due to the way their bodies manufacture and metabolize cholesterol, a difference due to heredity.

It's being realized increasingly that trans fatty acids, which include vegetable oils that are hydrogenated, increase the risk of heart disease. These are most commonly found in baked goods.

Balancing Your Cholesterol Levels

The government now requires that the presence of these substances be identified on the label.

Smoking also plays a role in cholesterol levels. Smokers tend to have a less healthy cholesterol balance.

HOW TO REACH YOUR
CHOLESTEROL GOALS

Trying to determine what your cholesterol goals are can be like trying to keep your eye on a moving target. The recommended cholesterol levels keep becoming more stringent. Furthermore, keep in mind that it's the way the components stack up that is important.

The American Heart Association recommends that all Americans have a total cholesterol level of less than 200 mg/dl, with 200–230 mg/dl considered "borderline undesirable" cholesterol, and undesirable cholesterol pegged at 240 mg/dl or higher. But, as a heart attack survivor, you're at higher risk for that next heart attack; therefore, you need to do better. In general, your total cholesterol level should be in the 160–170 mg/dl range. Your HDL cholesterol reading should be 40 mg/dl or higher, and your LDL cholesterol should be less than 100 mg/dl. Remember, the lower the LDL and the higher the HDL, the better. If you are at particularly high risk for another heart attack, or have had a very recent heart attack, your LDL goal is less than 70 mg/dl. Recently published guidelines recommend a target goal of less than 70 mg/dl for individuals at very high risk for a heart attack, even if they have never suffered a heart attack.

Sometimes a ratio instead of a number is used to explain the HDL cholesterol level. The ratio is obtained by dividing the HDL

Chapter Nine

cholesterol level into the total cholesterol number. If you have had a heart attack, a desirable range is 3.5 to 1. For instance, a total cholesterol of 180 and an HDL of 35 would result in a ratio of 5:1.

When it comes to triglycerides, your level should be less than 150 mg. This is also considered "desirable" by the American Heart Association. A borderline high triglyceride reading is 150–199 mg/dl, high is 200–400 mg/dl, and very high is 500 mg/dl or higher, they say.

Here are the top ways to reach your cholesterol goals:

- *Don't smoke:* Smoking decreases the HDL and increases LDL cholesterol levels.
- *Lose weight:* If you're overweight, you're more likely to have low HDL and high LDL and triglyceride levels. Weight loss can dramatically alter this, although it can take some time for the effect to become apparent.
- *Eat a cholesterol-smart diet:* Choose monounsaturated fats, like canola and olive oil, instead of saturated fat. This can lower your LDL cholesterol and improve your HDL cholesterol level without raising your total cholesterol number.
- *Exercise regularly:* Doing aerobic exercise especially raises HDL levels. You can raise your HDL by about a milligram for every four or five miles you walk each week. If that doesn't sound like much, remember, even modest HDL gains pay off.
- *Drink alcoholic beverages in moderation:* If you don't currently drink, taking up the habit to raise your HDL cholesterol is something that you may consider doing, in consultation with your doctor. If you are already a social

drinker, be assured that one or two ounces of alcohol a day can raise your HDL cholesterol by 5 to 10 percent.

HOW CHOLESTEROL DRUGS WORK

While it's best to have a high HDL cholesterol level and a low LDL cholesterol level, as of yet there are no medications that act solely to raise HDL cholesterol. So the key way to improve your cholesterol balance is to lower LDL cholesterol, and the top way to do that is with a type of drug known as "statins."

Indeed, statins have an ability to lower that LDL cholesterol number by 20–60 percent. They also have modest triglyceride-lowering and HDL-raising effects. This may be due to the previously mentioned seesaw effect, an effect explained by the complicated metabolism of these different lipid fractions, and the effect of medications on this metabolism. But the major impact of the statins is on LDL cholesterol, and they lower this type of cholesterol more than any other of the cholesterol-lowering drugs on the market. Pharmaceutical companies are racing to develop medications that preferentially raise HDL cholesterol.

NON-DRUG WAYS TO
BALANCE CHOLESTEROL

There are a number of reasons why some people should not—or will not—take cholesterol-lowering prescription drugs. The drugs may not suffice in helping them reach their goal cholesterol levels. Or they may only need to improve their cholesterol levels a small amount. Others may shy away from these drugs because they cannot tolerate the short-term adverse side effects, such as stomach distress. Some may develop one of the rare, serious side effects of the statins. Younger women may plan to become pregnant, so statin therapy is not appropriate.

Whatever the reason, there are some non-drug alternatives that can be quite effective in improving cholesterol levels. These include the following:

- *Polycosanol (policosanol):* Polycosanol is a mixture of fatty alcohols derived from the wax of honeybees or from sugar cane. It's been found that 10 mg per day can lower LDL cholesterol by 20 percent. Research, however, has not consistently demonstrated the benefit of polycosanol.
- *Plant sterols (phytosterols):* Plant steroids, and derivatives of them, known as plant sterols and stanols, are substances contained in small quantities in vegetable oils and such grains as corn, rye, and wheat. Structurally, they resemble cholesterol. If consumed in sufficient amount, they are absorbed in the body, and the amount of cholesterol absorbed by the digestive system is reduced. An easy way to consume enough sterols and stanols to result in this effect is to use "Benecol" or "Take Control" margarine. Two tablespoons of either of these can lower LDL cholesterol by 10–15 percent.
- *Flaxseed oil:* Like olive, canola, and most other plant oils, this rich oil that comes from the flax plant is unsaturated and heart healthy, because it contains alpha-linolenic acid. It can be purchased in tablet form. Taking 3–6 grams a day can lower LDL cholesterol by 15 percent.
- *Nuts:* Nuts are probably one of the easiest—and tastiest— ways to lower cholesterol. Eight walnuts a day can lower

LDL cholesterol by 22 percent, and 73 grams of almonds (a little over a half cup) can lower it by 9 percent.

- *Soy protein:* Soy protein, which is derived from the soybean plant, is rich in phytoestrogens, a natural form of estrogen, and alpha-linolenic acid, which converts into heart-protective omega-3 fatty acids. Sources of soy protein include tofu and dairy-substitute products made with soy. You can buy meat-substitute products made from soy to use in recipes, and soy flour for baking. Roasted soybeans are a good alternative to nuts. Eating 24 grams of soy protein a day can lower LDL cholesterol by 13 percent. For instance, 8 ounces of soymilk contain 4–10 grams, 4 ounces of tofu have 8–13 grams, 1 ounce of soy flour has 10–13 grams, and one-half cup of textured soy protein has about 11 grams of soy protein.

- *Fish oil:* Fish oil is rich in heart-protective omega-3 fatty acids, so you should eat fish, particularly fatty fish, at least two or three times a week. Taking fish oil capsules is a good way to get these substances as well, although whether you derive as much benefit from fish oil capsules instead of eating fish is unknown. \These are generally taken in a dosage of 3 grams a day. Larger doses of fish oil (8–12 grams a day) can lower triglycerides by 20–30 percent, but this dosage should be used only under a doctor's supervision because of potential side effects. Fish oil in large doses is used to lower triglycerides; it does not generally lower total cholesterol.

- *Fiber:* Fiber, which is the indigestible part of fruits, vegetables, and grains, has no nutritional value in itself, but it can lower cholesterol. Fiber falls into two general categories—water soluble (found mostly in oats, fruit, and legumes) and water insoluble (found mostly in grains and vegetables). Both are beneficial, but it is the soluble type that is credited with lowering cholesterol. To get this effect, you should consume 10–25 grams a day. Using oats as filler in casseroles and meat loaf will help you consume this type of fiber. Lentils can be eaten as a side dish or made into soup, and peanuts make a tasty snack. Starting our day by eating oatmeal is a terrific idea.

In short, there are a lot of ways to improve your cholesterol balance. And since this is a key means of reducing your risk of having another heart attack, this is something you should get started on immediately.

TEN

Your Three-Part Program for Heart Attack Prevention

This book contains many tips to help you prevent another heart attack, such as how to work with your doctor, how to make sure you take your medications properly, and how to get help in an emergency. But one major thing you need to do for yourself is to be on a three-pronged program for heart attack prevention. This three-part program is not easy—each of the three components requires major lifestyle changes. But these are the steps you must take to tackle the root causes of atherosclerosis, the progressive coronary artery disease that sets the stage for your heart attack in the first place.

These three steps are:

1. *Quit smoking:* If you smoke, you must stop, to protect your heart.
2. *Exercise:* Becoming physically active is important to protect your heart.
3. *Adopt a heart-healthy diet:* Eating the right food can protect your heart.

Chapter Ten

These three steps are the cornerstone to speed your recovery from a heart attack, and they can also keep your future as heart attack free as possible.

PART ONE: QUIT SMOKING

Smoking is among the toughest habits to kick, but if you are a heart attack survivor who smokes, quitting is your Number One priority. Smoking is one of the four "super" risk factors and contributes to a whopping 80 percent of heart attacks. That's what research has found. But you don't need research to discover the pivotal role that smoking plays in heart attacks. Just drop by a cardiac care unit and chat with the patients there. You'll soon be convinced!

That said, though, quitting is one of the hardest things you'll ever do. Just because it's the most worthwhile doesn't mean it's going to be easy. The important thing, though, is that it's doable—and you're going to do it!

1. Learn the Facts About Smoking

Here is mental ammunition to help you quit. You may know some of these facts; others you may not. Commit them to your memory and tell them to yourself as often as possible. Keep in mind that:

- Women smokers are up to five times more likely to suffer a heart attack than are women non-smokers.
- Smoking as few as four cigarettes a day raises your heart attack risk.
- Cigarettes contain toxic chemicals that damage the walls of your coronary arteries, setting the stage for a heart attack.

■ Tobacco smoke makes your blood more likely to clot, and blood clots ultimately cause heart attacks.

These dangers exist even if you smoke "low-tar" and "low-nicotine" cigarettes, a cigar, or a pipe. Oral contraceptives raise heart attack risk when used by smokers. Both oral contraceptives and tobacco contain blood-clotting properties. This can spell disaster for a heart attack survivor.

Smoking marijuana is also dangerous to your heart, especially in middle-aged people, because it increases the amount of oxygen your heart needs. This can spark a heart attack, especially in heart attack survivors, who most likely have some form of coronary artery disease.

---

12 STEPS TO QUIT SMOKING

Stopping the cigarette habit is easier said than done, so we're going to help you formulate your own 12-step plan to quit smoking. Here's a rundown:

1. Learn the facts about smoking.
2. Formulate a quit-smoking plan.
3. Team up with a buddy.
4. Consider nicotine replacement or anti-smoking medication.
5. Look into Stop Smoking programs.
6. Consider counseling.
7. Stock your refrigerator with healthy foods.
8. Cut your caffeine intake in half.
9. Create "stress busters."
10. Take advantage of cardiac rehab.
11. Be prepared to backslide.
12. Reward yourself.

Chapter Ten

Also, women who smoke are more vulnerable to heart-attack-causing spasms of the coronary arteries.

Smoking is a proven health hazard. As a heart attack survivor, protecting your heart should be your top concern. But it's not only your heart that is damaged by smoking. Here are the other leading killers and disabling diseases of women linked to smoking. This makes tobacco-related diseases the leading cause of preventable deaths in women:

- Lung cancer
- Cervical cancer
- Colon cancer
- Osteoporosis
- Stroke—and as a heart attack survivor, you're already at increased risk of stroke

2. Formulate a Plan

You have plenty of reasons to quit smoking, but the question remains: how do you do it? It's estimated that 73 percent of women smokers want to quit but don't because they are addicted. There's some evidence that women may be even more strongly addicted to smoking than are men. So, if you find quitting difficult, seek solutions. Don't spend fruitless time beating yourself up emotionally over it.

Smoking is an exceptionally difficult addiction to overcome because it is not only a physiological addiction but a psychological one as well. It is an ingrained habit, which is done with behavioral cues—like having a cigarette with that first cup of coffee at breakfast, or while watching television at night.

The effects of nicotine are fast, predictable, and reliable, and you can get them virtually on demand. So you're going to need all the help you can to achieve your goal of turning your back on your seemingly friendly cigarette, which really is the deadliest of enemies in disguise.

It's important to have a plan in place before you try to quit. This helps because you can anticipate the obstacles that may arise and map a strategy ahead of time to overcome them.

Make sure that you make quitting smoking your Number One priority. Sometimes women smoke to control their weight. About an estimated 20 percent of women don't gain weight if they try to quit, but the majority gain 5–15 pounds. A very tiny majority may put on more than that, but this is highly unusual. If you are looking to substitute one risk for another as an excuse to keep smoking, don't look to us. If you smoke and you need to lose weight, put off the weight part temporarily, because it is smoking that poses the greater danger to your heart. By quitting smoking, you may gain a small amount of weight, but this will be more than offset by the decrease in heart attack risk that you'll reap.

When it comes to formulating a plan, you also need to choose the right time—and the right strategy—to quit. Your hormones may play a role in your success in quitting. Women who try to quit right before or during their menstrual period may experience worse withdrawal symptoms. In addition, some women crave cigarettes right before they get their period, so this obviously is not the best time during the month to quit. A better choice might be a few days after your period.

You also need to prepare for your "quit day," should that be the strategy you choose. You may have friends who brag that they quit "cold turkey." If you can do this, great. But don't be disheartened

Chapter Ten

if you cannot—most research shows this is very difficult to do. Some smoking cessation programs encourage a technique known as "nicotine fading," in which smokers switch over to cigarette brands progressively lower in tar and nicotine. You can make preparations, such as working out a schedule that outlines how you'll gradually be decreasing the number of cigarettes you're smoking, deciding on stress busters, or as you will see in the next step, lining up a quitting "buddy."

3. Team Up

Finding a friend who sincerely wants to quit smoking to buddy up with can be very valuable, just as dieting with a friend can be. Your buddy may be your spouse or a friend who also needs to quit. Even if you don't have such a partner, there are other options; you can find other people who want to quit smoking at a smoking cessation program, or check the Internet for support groups in cyberspace.

You might consider asking your quitting buddy to join you in a friendly wager, to see which of you can succeed in becoming an ex-smoker. If there's a tie, you both win!

4. Consider Nicotine Replacement or Medication

It's not surprising that people become dependent on smoking, because nicotine increases the levels of certain chemicals, such as dopamine and norepinephrine, in the brain. These chemicals can give you a lift, but the downside is that, when you try to quit smoking and their levels drop, this can cause withdrawal symptoms. It is estimated that up to 80 percent of people may experience withdrawal symptoms. Such symptoms can be intense for two or three

---

THE MOST COMMON WITHDRAWAL SYMPTOMS

- Depression
- Insomnia
- Irritability
- Frustration or anger
- Anxiety
- Difficulty concentrating
- Restlessness

---

days, but within 10 to 14 days after quitting, most usually subside. Still, in order to quit, many people need help—in the form of nicotine replacement, other medication, or a combination of both. If you're one of the many women who are bothered by withdrawal symptoms, a nicotine substitute or non-nicotine medication may help immensely.

You may wonder, since nicotine is harmful to your heart, why nicotine substitutes are touted. There's good reason for this. First, nicotine replacement products supply the body with less of the substance: about one-third to one-half the amount found in most cigarettes. This makes it less harmful. Second, although they contain nicotine, these products do not contain many of the other toxic chemicals also present in cigarettes. Third, you're using them with a goal in mind—that of quitting smoking. And that is very healthful. But, as a heart attack survivor, you should consult with your doctor before using these products. And never smoke while using a nicotine substitute, such as a patch. That megadose of nicotine can prove dangerous to your heart.

Which type of nicotine replacement is best? The one that appeals to you most and, therefore, you are most likely to use. There are now a number of different types of nicotine replacement aids on the market.

Nicotine gum is available over the counter. The gum releases small amounts of nicotine, which is absorbed by the body and cuts down on withdrawal symptoms. A nicotine patch is another way to administer nicotine and delivers the drug through your skin in a gradual fashion. Over time (months), the strength of the patch is gradually decreased. Nicotine replacement is also available in a nasal spray, oral lozenges, and an oral inhaler.

As with any drug, all of these products have side effects, but these are generally mild, such as stomach upset, coughing, or throat irritation, depending on the replacement method you choose. If you find yourself too bothered by these side effects, stop using that form and try another one.

An alternative to nicotine replacement is a prescription medication known as bupropion (Zyban.) This drug, marketed in another form as an antidepressant, boosts the levels of those brain chemicals mentioned earlier, dopamine and norepinephrine, the same way in which nicotine does.

This medication is generally prescribed for people who prefer a non-nicotine product or for those who have tried nicotine replacement products without success. Studies find that using this drug also doubles the chances of quitting. It can also be particularly helpful if you become depressed when you try to quit. Using this medication together with a nicotine replacement system may further increase the success of quitting compared to your success with either drug alone.

A newer anti-smoking medication, varenicline tartrate (Chantix) contains no nicotine but is unique because it is specifically designed to partially activate the nicotinic receptor and reduce the severity of the smoker's craving and the withdrawal symptoms. Moreover, if a person smokes a cigarette while receiving treatment, Chantix has the potential to diminish the sense of satisfaction associated with smoking. This may help to break the cycle of nicotine addiction.

According to the research, using nicotine replacement or anti-smoking medication doubles your chance of quitting. But you can bolster this effect by combining using a product with counseling, or enrolling in a formal smoking cessation program to increase your probability of success.

If you've tried to quit before and found it very tough, you may need to use both bupropion and a nicotine replacement product to be successful this time. But this should only be done under a doctor's supervision.

5. Look into Stop Smoking Programs

To increase your chances of successfully giving up cigarettes, consider a formal smoking cessation program. You can use a program alone or in combination with nicotine replacement or anti-smoking medication.

A number of organizations, including the American Heart Association, the American Lung Association, the American Cancer Society, and the Seventh Day Adventists, sponsor effective anti-smoking programs. You may also check your local hospital, the Yellow pages, adult education programs, and your local "Y", church, or synagogue. Excellent programs abound. The types of programs can vary; check them out and find one that suits you.

6. Consider Counseling

Smoking is a very tough addiction; there's no sense toughing it out by yourself if you don't need to. Some women who are clinically depressed or who suffer from anxiety disorder find that smoking helps keep these symptoms at bay. For these women, it may be especially difficult to quit smoking. If you think you may be in this group, consider getting additional help, such as psychological counseling or medication, before you try to quit smoking.

7. Stock Your Refrigerator with Healthful Foods

Pay attention to nutrition. While dieting can be difficult during this time, concentrating on fruits, vegetables, and high-fiber foods that are filling can be useful. One study on quitting smoking found that eating several small meals throughout the day helped keep the participants' blood sugar levels stable, lessening their cravings. Low-fat "comfort" foods like fat-free chocolate pudding can also help.

8. Cut Your Caffeine Intake in Half

Some smoking cessation programs advise completely cutting out caffeine, particularly coffee, reasoning that, since so many people smoke and drink coffee at the same time, this helps break the habit. But caffeine, like nicotine, is also a stimulant with addictive qualities, and quitting can bring on withdrawal symptoms, including severe headache, which can also be unbearable. If you experience this, decrease your caffeine intake slowly, until you've halved it.

9. Create "Stress Busters"

Many women smoke as a way to manage stress. Choosing a stress management technique, like yoga or meditation, can be very helpful. Also, many women find they need "to do something with their hands" to take the place of cigarettes. Knitting, hooking rugs, and needlepoint are alternatives. Just be certain you find these activities enjoyable, not stress producing.

10. Take Advantage of Cardiac Rehabilitation

If you go to a cardiac rehabilitation class that offers smoking cessation help, go for it! Getting involved in both cardiac rehab and quitting smoking will pay off big dividends in heart protection. For more on cardiac rehabilitation, see Part Two of the program, later in this chapter.

11. Be Prepared to Backslide

You are most likely to begin smoking again in the first few weeks after quitting. If you are aware of this danger period, you are more likely to be able to resist having "just one cigarette." But even if you relapse, this doesn't mean you're a permanent failure. Even if you relapse and smoke an entire cigarette during the first week, you're not necessarily doomed. Studies show that such slips are a normal part of "learning to quit." And remember, most people who successfully quit have failed at least once, and maybe more!

12. Reward Yourself

Becoming a non-smoker pays off big and is certainly a reward in itself. But don't forget to reward yourself along the way! Set up milestones—honor yourself for going a day, then a week, and then a month without a cigarette. Pamper yourself, buy yourself a little treat, and make quitting a cause for celebration. You can bankroll these goodies by using the money that you would have

Chapter Ten

spent on cigarettes. Just set aside a special jar for the cash, and watch the dollars mount up.

PART TWO: EXERCISE FOR YOUR HEART

Before your heart attack, you were either an exercise enthusiast, a couch potato, or most likely somewhere in between. That was before. Now, you no longer have an option. You are going to exercise regularly; it's a requirement that must be followed as religiously as taking your cardiovascular medication, if you want to stay heart attack free. But the best thing is that an exercise program is good for the mind, body, and soul—and it's fun.

The Benefits of Exercise

Although the heart is referred to as a muscle, exercise does not specifically strengthen it. But exercise and conditioning help the entire cardiovascular system function more effectively and efficiently. This system includes the pump (the heart) and the plumbing (arteries and veins). Exercise makes the parts of the system work in better harmony, which in turn makes your cardiovascular system function more efficiently.

- Regular exercise promotes the formation of new blood vessels. These new vessels, known as collateral vessels, bring blood to the heart, despite blockages in your coronary arteries. They also contribute additional blood flow to areas not receiving an ample supply of blood due to damaged or scarred tissue from a heart attack.
- Exercise impacts major heart attack risk factors. Exercise can dramatically improve blood pressure. If you're on blood pressure medication, you may be able to reduce it

through regular exercise. If you have "borderline" high blood pressure, you may be able to eliminate the need for medication.

- Exercise dramatically affects diabetes. When you exercise, your body uses insulin more efficiently. This is tremendously important—it means that, if you've been told you are "insulin resistant" (pre-diabetic), physical exercise and losing weight may save you from developing diabetes. If you are already diabetic, exercise may help you cut down on your medication.
- Exercise helps balance cholesterol levels. It can help raise your HDL (or "good") cholesterol, especially when your triglycerides are elevated.
- As if that wasn't enough, exercise is good not only for your heart but the rest of your body as well. Exercise is believed to help reduce the risk for several types of cancer, including colon cancer. Also, exercise is very beneficial for building bone mass, which helps prevent osteoporosis, the "bone-thinning disease" of elder women.
- Exercise helps you lose weight, be more alert, sleep better, and stay in a good mood, thereby promoting self-esteem.

In short, exercise is *all* good.

Cardiac Rehabilitation

What's the best exercise for a heart attack survivor, and how do you get started on an exercise program? Cardiac rehabilitation is the answer.

Cardiac rehabilitation is a structured, supervised program of exercise, education, and emotional support. The program can

Chapter Ten

benefit you whether you were an ardent fitness buff before your heart attack, or you hadn't gotten near a gym since high school. Age doesn't matter either; everyone works at her own level.

It also doesn't matter how severe a heart attack you had. This program will benefit you if your heart attack was mild and without complications, or if you suffered a more severe one that left your heart damaged. Cardiac rehab can benefit women with congestive heart failure and with some types of heartbeat irregularities, such as those that occur during exercise. You can even exercise in a cardiac rehab program if you have an implanted defibrillator. In fact, even if you are physically disabled, cardiac rehab can still work for you.

One of the best things about cardiac rehab is that it helps you regain your confidence in your physical abilities. After a heart attack, one of the most common fears is that physical exertion will bring on another one. In a cardiac rehab program, you get to test out your physical abilities in a safe environment monitored by trained cardiac professionals.

There are three stages to cardiac rehabilitation. You may undergo the first phase without even realizing it. This occurs while you're in the hospital. A cardiac rehab therapist will visit you and teach you some exercises. You'll also be given an exercise program to continue at home: probably some warm-up exercises and walking. Before you know it, you'll probably be walking a couple of miles a day.

Then, once you're home, you can enroll in the second phase, which involves traveling to an outpatient cardiac rehab center. This might be at your hospital, another hospital nearby, or in a freestanding clinic. It may look like a regular fitness center, but there are some important differences. This is usually seen in the amount of attention you're given. You'll be taught to use each piece of equipment properly, and while you exercise, your heart will be monitored. This information also may be shared with your doctor, who can use it to see if any of the medication you're on needs to be adjusted, for example.

Once you graduate from this phase, you can go on to phase three, in which you either continue to exercise in the cardiac rehab program indefinitely, or you excercise in a fitness center. Some women prefer the supportive environment of the cardiac rehab facility; others choose to join a fitness center, or go back to their regular one. Whichever option you choose is up to you; the important thing is that you continue your program of regular exercise.

All cardiac rehab programs have physical exercise as their focus, but some offer additional educational programs as well. These additional components vary, but they can include information on smoking cessation, nutrition, medication, diabetes and high blood pressure, stress management, and more. If you need to tackle some lifestyle changes—such as quitting smoking or learning to manage your diabetes—look for a cardiac rehab program that offers these classes. For instance, if you need to make major changes in the way you eat, you may need the help of a dietician—not just someone who will teach you for a few sessions, but an expert who will really pay attention to you. Think back to when you were in school, when you needed to master a difficult subject, like calculus. It was easier to do so with a tutor. A dietician can help you master nutrition in much the same way. But perhaps the most valuable component of cardiac rehab for many women is the emotional support you'll receive.

To find the cardiac rehab program that's best for you, you may need to shop around. Talk to your doctor about what is available at the hospital where you were treated, but also don't hesitate to call elsewhere and talk to the cardiac rehab director.

Chapter Ten

Above all, don't let anything deter you from cardiac rehab. As with exercising on your own (which we'll get to in a moment), it's easy to find lots of reasons to postpone—sometimes indefinitely—getting into a cardiac rehab program. First, there's the cost. It's true that cardiac rehab may be too expensive for people who do not have health insurance. But fortunately, Medicare and many types of insurance and managed care plans will pay for cardiac rehab, especially in the case of heart attack survivors. And, for most people, cardiac rehab often costs less than joining a gym.

Then, there's the time factor. You may have time for cardiac rehab when you've got time off from work for recuperation. But what will happen when you go back to work? Well, the truth is that, whether it's cardiac rehab or not, you're still going to have to carve out time for a regular exercise program, no matter what kind it is.

Don't be turned off if you peer into the cardiac rehab area and see only men exercising there. Traditionally, cardiac rehab programs have attracted more men than women. At least in the past, doctors were less likely to refer women to cardiac rehabilitation programs, even if they were good candidates. So it's not surprising that the enrollment in cardiac rehab tends to be male dominated. But women of all ages are very welcome in cardiac rehab programs, so don't let anything deter you from benefiting from this valuable program.

Take Carmen, a 58-year-old heart attack survivor who admitted she was a little skeptical when she realized that the men outnumbered the women in her program. But now, two years after her heart attack, she's a regular, going three times a week after work.

"The guys boost you up here; it's good for your morale," Carmen notes. "I got to know the guys after a while and we all kid around with each other."

Creating Your Custom Exercise Program

In an ideal world, every heart patient who could benefit from a cardiac rehab program would enroll in it. But this is not always feasible for everyone. Happily, even if you cannot—or choose not to—participate in cardiac rehab, you can still reap the same benefit from exercising on your own, providing that you do the exercises properly and stick with them.

The best way to create your own program, or "exercise prescription," is to work one out with your doctor. Your doctor can help you create a plan that is tailored for you by taking a number of factors into consideration, including your age, your condition, and the results of your exercise stress tests.

Your heart rate is the barometer, which can tell the intensity with which you are exercising. The more intense the exercise, the higher your heart rate. Your exercise prescription, for instance, may instruct you to raise your heart rate to a specific level and then maintain it for a certain amount of time—say, 20 minutes—and then cool down gradually. It is when your heart is working at this sustained level that you are reaping the benefits of exercise.

Your doctor will show you ways that you can monitor your heart rate to ensure that you are working at the right intensity. There are various ways to do this. Heart monitors, which you can wear like a wristwatch, are becoming increasingly popular. You can also gauge your exercise intensity by monitoring your pulse rate. If you do not know how to do so already, your doctor or the office nurse can show you how to take your own pulse. For instance, your program may call for you to exercise until your pulse gets to a certain rate and then maintain that intensity for about 20 minutes. This figure is usually 70–80 percent of the maximum pulse rate you achieved during your exercise stress test. You'll then be told to cool down for the remaining time to get your pulse back to its normal level.

Checking your pulse rate periodically as you exercise is the most accurate way to monitor your intensity. You can also monitor your perception of how vigorously you are working by using the method known as the Borg Scale. The Borg Scale is a simple rating of perceived exertion (RPE). Many coaches and physiologists use this method to assess an athlete's level of intensity during training or testing sessions. There are different types of scales used, but the 20-point one is common. Number one is sitting, but the scale starts at 6, because that is very, very light exercise, and it goes to 20, which is so intense that you can do it about four minutes before you have to quit in total exhaustion. Most people exercise at about 14–16, which is the moderately hard to hard range.

To exercise using the Borg Scale, you warm up for 15–20 minutes, then vigorously exercise on a bicycle or treadmill to the point where you almost have to quit for a couple of minutes. That is your "20" point of exertion. Then you slow your rate of exertion for a cooling-down period. This method can also be done using a 15-point scale; it all depends on the type of scale that your doctor prefers. You should not exercise at a full "20" level without your doctor's permission.

How much exercise do you need to protect your heart? This is a common question people always ask. It's human nature to want to know exactly how much exercise—or what type of exercise—is most beneficial. There's a lot of confusion about this, because contradictory studies are always being published about it. What's important to remember is that, no matter what the studies say, they never challenge the principle that exercise is very beneficial.

Of course, how fast you work up to your typical exercise program will depend on your physical condition. Generally, you should exercise at least two hours a week, breaking this down into four half-hour sessions. But remember, work up to this level at the pace which your doctor recommends. And, in the case of exercise, less is not more. More is best.

You may wonder why you need a program of regular exercise if you already have an active routine and are always dashing from meeting to meeting, or running errands, or hurrying to pick up the kids at school. But this is different. Working out on a treadmill or bicycle for 30 minutes daily makes your heart pump better and more efficiently. If you go dancing, garden, or play golf once a week, that's fine, but you also need to exercise in a way that is going to make your heart beat faster than what it normally would for a set period of time in order to benefit.

The Three Types of Exercise You Need

When you think of heart-healthy exercise, you probably think automatically of an aerobics class. That's necessary for sound cardiovascular health, of course. But you also need flexibility and strength. This will not only help you strengthen your entire body but will also build in variety. And variety adds the spice that will keep you exercising. So here are the components to help build your program:

- *Aerobic exercise:* Aerobics are a sustained form of exercise during which your heartbeat remains in an elevated range for a sustained period of time. Aerobic activities include brisk walking, jogging, swimming, pool aerobics, bicycling, dancing, calisthenics, racquet sports, using free weights and pulleys, and using rowing and skiing machines.

- *Strengthening exercise:* Also known as resistance training, this type of exercise provides impact on your joints and, in doing so, stimulates the ends of your bones. This type of exercise strengthens you, helps ward off osteoporosis, and helps you lose weight. Strengthening exercises include working with weights, either free weights or machines.

- *Stretching exercise:* Stretching promotes flexibility, which is a very important component of a well-rounded exercise program. This type of exercise provides increased flexibility around your joints, which prevents injury. But stretching has other benefits. It feels great and helps alleviate stress. You can increase your flexibility by doing simple stretching exercises for your legs, lower back, calves, arms, shoulders, chest, and neck. Programs such as yoga and tai chi promote flexibility.

Exercise Tips

Okay, we all know that exercise is important—and for you, the heart attack survivor, imperative. So why are you still unenthusiastic? "Lack of time" is the main reason many people cite, followed by "It's boring." Here's a list of tips to convince you otherwise:

- *Build in variety:* Don't do the same thing every session. If you dislike exercising on a treadmill, don't do it. Take a brisk walk outdoors instead. Ride a bicycle, jump rope, swim, go dancing—do whatever makes your heart beat faster, not only with exercise but enjoyment as well.

- *Vary your exercise program according to the seasons:* You need to find a way to exercise year-round, whether you do so at home, the gym, at work, outdoors in good weather, or at a mall walking club if it's rainy. Don't use the excuse that it's too hot or too cold; you can find an exercise activity to suit any climate. There are two very cheap and easy ways to exercise. If it's nice out, walk out the door and turn right (or left) and keep on walking. If it's bad weather, or if you're stuck at work, use the stairs as your exercise machinery. If you've got a 15-minute break, take 5 minutes for your coffee, then spend the next 10 walking up and down the stairs.
- *Make exercise fun:* Join a gym and make new friends there. Pick a facility in which you feel comfortable. Or round up your spouse or some friends. That way, if you fall off the exercise wagon—if you get a cold or miss some sessions for another reason—you'll have a support group clamoring for you to come back.
- *Try something new:* With the exercise business booming, there is no lack of new types of classes and exercises to try out. Pilates may be hot, but spinning is not. Who knows what the latest exercise fad will be? As long as they follow sound principles, all exercise programs work.
- *Pay attention to your body clock:* If you're a morning person, do your exercise when you first awaken. If you're a night person, you might prefer exercising later in the day or before you go to bed.
- *Increase your activity level gradually:* If you're doing a mile on a treadmill, don't add another mile all at once. Start by adding a quarter of a mile. Continue for a few

weeks at this new level, then add another quarter of a mile, and so on.

- *Safety first:* Always make sure you stay in well-populated areas. If a walk through the woods suits you, bring a friend. If you use a gym at night, make sure the parking lot is well lit.

Tips for Women 65 or Older

If you are 65 or older, your body needs exercise just as it did when you were younger. But you may need to choose different exercises than when you were younger. Here are some guidelines:

- Minimize the possibility of injury by choosing low-impact activities instead of high-impact ones. Low-impact activities include walking, biking, swimming, rowing, cross-country skiing, stair-climbing, and low-impact aerobics. You can reap the same cardiovascular benefits from exercising longer at a lower intensity that you can from a shorter, more vigorous workout. If you have physical limitations, such as poor vision, poor balance, or conditions that affect your ability to exercise, such as arthritis, work with your doctor to find the most appropriate activities.

- Aim for slow and steady progress. Remember, exercise is important for everyone, but for you, as a heart attack survivor, it is imperative. You must exercise regularly to protect your heart. Also, although good medical care can guide you through your recuperation, it is only through exercise that you can achieve a level of fitness and well-being that will equal, or even surpass, the way you were before you had your heart attack.

PART THREE: EAT HEART SMART

The third component in your Three-Part Program for Heart Attack Prevention is as close as your refrigerator. Eating healthy is important for your heart, especially if you're overweight. If you weigh more than you should, your heart attack risk is increased. You're also at risk of developing—or worsening—one of the major heart attack risk factors: high blood pressure, unhealthy cholesterol levels, and diabetes.

On the other hand, if you're slender but have lousy eating habits, you're not doing your heart—or your overall health—any good. Too often, it's only the overweight person who is looked upon as a potential heart attack patient. But that isn't always the case, as many slender heart attack survivors can attest. So there are a lot of reasons to eat heart smart, no matter what your scale reads.

What Is Heart-Smart Eating?

What does eating smart for your heart really mean? Over the years, this concept has changed and, thankfully, for the better. Just a few years ago, eating heart smart meant downing meals that were low in fat but also low in taste as well. Broiled dry fish. Chalky plain baked potatoes. Salads suited more for rabbits than for red-blooded women. Nowadays, there are ways to create meals that are not only good for you but taste good too. Heart-smart eating is now much more appealing.

The accent, though, is on the word "smart," because you have to be smart about the way you chose your foods. Also take note of the word "strategy." That's the way we like to look at it. "Diets" don't work. Never did, and most likely never will. But using a heart-smart strategy to create a healthy way to eat is a different story.

The Truth About Losing Weight

Our weight-loss folklore is based on fads and fallacies, not grounded in facts. To become leaner is to ignore much of what our weight-obsessed culture endeavors to teach about nutrition, because often what is passed off as nutritional advice has more to do with eating fads, not science. But here are some suggestions that can provide you with a more realistic approach to paring off the pounds.

Be realistic about what you see in the mirror. Your body type is determined by genetics. This doesn't mean you can't modify your body somewhat, but you should be realistic. Feeling bad about the way you look will not make you eat less; it will only make you eat more.

Work steadily and patiently toward your weight-loss goal. Miracle fast weight-loss diets have as much chance of succeeding in the long run as, say, encountering an actual miracle. It took a while for that weight to appear, and it will take a while for it to disappear.

All diets work for a little time and then fail. This is why it's important to make lifelong changes in the way you eat.

Why Diets Don't Work

The first diet in book form was popularized over a century ago, and diet books haven't stopped flying off the bookstore shelves yet. Yet many Americans are fatter than ever. Why is this so?

Your Three-Part Program for Heart Attack Prevention

Many diet books have two things in common:

1. They promise weight loss without changing habits or employing discipline.
2. Whatever food plan they promulgate is too restrictive to stick to on a daily basis, year in and year out.

All diets work for a while and, ultimately, all diets fail. This leads to a phenomenon known as "yo-yo dieting," with which you may be all too familiar. This cycling way of taking off pounds and putting them back on again is, in addition to being demoralizing, dangerous to your health. Studies find that, eventually, all the weight is gained back. Not only that, it can also have a bad effect on your cholesterol levels.

Everything in moderation is best. The best way to eat heart smart is to avoid food plans that stress one type of food over another. Most foods can be enjoyed in moderation. Consider red meat, for example. For years, this food was considered a red flag when it came to heart-healthy eating, and it is probably still a good idea to avoid that thick, well-marbled steak. But lean beef, which is rich in protein, phosphorous, zinc, and B-complex vitamins, can be eaten in moderation.

Or consider chocolate. Any diet guru who is going to tell a woman to give up chocolate is going to be a loser from the start. Research finds dark chocolate may have health-providing properties, including phenols, the antioxidant chemicals also present in wine, which can help prevent heart disease. A host of research shows that wine, particularly the red variety, may have health-providing properties. This doesn't mean you should go out and create a diet of steak, chocolate, and red wine. But it does speak to the fact that most foods—even those previously thought forbidden—can be enjoyed in moderation.

Heart-Smart Eating—Mediterranean Style

The Mediterranean diet—which is not really a diet but a lifestyle—is advocated by Dr. Walter Willett and his colleagues at the Harvard School of Public Health. Here's how it works:

1. *Carbohydrates:* Eat carbohydrates at most meals, but in the form of whole grains, including oatmeal, whole-wheat bread, and brown rice. The body cannot metabolize whole grains as quickly as it processes "white" foods (white bread, white rice, and potatoes), and that delay keeps blood sugar and insulin levels from rising too quickly, which will keep you from getting hungry. So, if it's "white," avoid it.

2. *Oils and fats:* You can consume these without limits as long as they are healthy unsaturated fats, such as olive, canola, soy, corn, sunflower, peanut, and other vegetable oils. Steer clear of foods containing partially hydrogenated vegetable oil and trans-fatty acids. Trans-fatty acids are a type of saturated fat that is particularly bad for your heart, and they are found in many processed foods. Become a label reader and ferret them out.

3. *Fruits and vegetables:* These can and should be enjoyed in abundance. Fruits should be eaten two or three times a day. A diet rich in fruits and vegetables guards against heart attacks and strokes.

4. *Fish, poultry, and eggs:* Eat these up to twice a day. Eating fish can reduce the risk of heart disease. Chicken and turkey are also good lean sources of protein, low in saturated fat.

5. *Nuts and legumes:* These are excellent sources of protein, fiber, vitamins, and minerals, and they can be eaten one to three times daily. Legumes include black beans, navy beans, garbanzo beans, and other beans that are usually sold dry. Many kinds of nuts contain healthy fats, and some, such as walnuts and almonds, can lower cholesterol.

6. *Dairy products:* Dairy products, including milk and cheese, contain calcium, which is important for strong bones. Choose low-fat varieties, though, or take a calcium supplement with vitamin D.

7. *Red meat and butter:* These should be eaten sparingly, because they are high in saturated fat.

8. *Starches and sugars:* White rice, white bread, potatoes, and sweets aren't forbidden (which is one of the things we like about this approach to healthy eating), but they should be eaten only sparingly.

Low-Carbohydrate and Other Diets

In recent years, the South Beach Diet, advocated by Dr. Arthur Agatston, and the Atkins Diet, advocated by the late Dr. Robert Atkins, have skyrocketed in popularity. These and other low-carb diets are based on eschewing simple carbohydrates (those "white" foods again, like white rice, white pasta, and white bread) in favor of complex carbohydrates. Sugar is also considered a "no-no." Both diets start with a very carb-restrictive, two-week introductory phase. But while the Atkins diet is renowned for including foods like bacon, steak, and whole cheese, Agatston's plan takes an approach that is lower in saturated fat. Both plans eventually incorporate limited amounts of whole grains. Fruits, which are high in natural sugar, are severely limited, as are starchy veggies.

When the Atkins diet first become popular, the American Medical Association accused Dr. Atkins of risking the health of Americans. But the health risks never materialized, and in recent years, short-term studies find it improves cholesterol levels. This is largely due to the fact that people do lose weight, although initially much of this is water weight.

There are lots of other diet choices out there. Weight Watchers now incorporates both the traditional low-fat eating, called the Flex Plan, and a less restrictive plan based on low-carb foods, called the Core Plan. The Core Plan incorporates the use of whole grains and pasta.

When you look beneath the surface, there are some striking similarities to these plans. After the restrictive two-week period, when grains are added back to the low-carb plans, they generally specify whole grains, along with fresh fruits and vegetables. "White" foods, such as white rice and foods made with white flour, are usually included sparingly, if at all.

There is also the DASH diet, also discussed in this book, and the diet promulgated by Dr. Dean Ornish, which also has been found, in clinical studies, to reduce the risk of heart attacks. If you don't like to eat meat, you may find the latter plan suits you, as only 10 percent of calories are allowed from fat, which basically makes this a vegetarian diet as well. Plant-based foods that are high in fat are excluded, including all oils, nuts, and avocados. So it's basically fruits, vegetables, grains, and beans that compose most of the diet, supplemented by moderate amounts of non-fat dairy and egg whites.

Heart-Smart Eating Tips

So, what do you eat to stay healthy? For one thing, there is no one "best" way to eat, no matter what all the diet bestsellers proclaim. The best food strategy is the one that will work for you. As we noted earlier, we find that the Mediterranean diet's Healthy Eating Pyramid has a lot of appeal. Virtually every type of food is incorporated; the diet is low in saturated fat, made palatable by the liberal allowance of plant-based oil, and rich in fruits and vegetables. There is also a growing body of scientific evidence that backs it up. If you're zeroing in on high blood pressure, give the DASH diet a try. If Weight Watchers appeals to you, these diets are quite well balanced. And, if you're very disciplined, or you want a vegetarian diet, the Ornish diet may be the way to go.

In the meanwhile, though, here are tips you can use to create a Heart-Smart Eating Strategy of your own.

1. Cut back on saturated fat.

When it comes to dietary fats, all of them contain the same number of calories, but they differ widely in their effect on our body. Saturated fat raises blood cholesterol more than does anything else you can eat. Examples of saturated fats include butter, lard, meat fat, shortening, and hydrogenated oils such as palm and coconut oil, palm kernel oil, and cocoa butter. Stay away from trans-fatty acids as well. Stick to the plant-based fats, like olive oil, canola oil, or monounsaturated vegetable oil.

2. Replenish your supply of calcium daily.

Your Number One goal is to prevent another heart attack, but that doesn't mean you should neglect your bones. Since it's difficult to get enough calcium from the foods you eat, you should take a daily calcium supplement—1,000 mg of calcium prior to menopause and 1,500 mg if you're past menopause.

Chapter Ten

3. Eat plenty of fruits and vegetables.

Eating at least five daily servings of both fruits and vegetables each day may lower the risk of coronary heart disease, cancer, and possibly stroke as well. Fruits and vegetables are loaded with antioxidant vitamins, including beta carotene (which the body converts to vitamin A), vitamin E, and vitamin C. Foods containing antioxidants can help protect against heart disease. In addition, there's evidence that fruits and vegetables contain scores of micronutrients that may protect against cancer. Here are some particulars:

- *Vitamin C:* Broccoli, brussels sprouts, cantaloupe, cauliflower, currants (fresh), mango, peppers, kiwi, papayas, oranges, parsley strawberries, red cabbages, and grapefruit.
- *Vitamin E:* Dried apricots, mango, pumpkin seeds, fortified cereals, sweet potatoes, wheat germ, sunflower seeds, asparagus, and raw kale.
- *Vitamin A:* Broccoli, carrots, sweet potatoes, pumpkin, yellow squash, cooked spinach, tomatoes, kale, red peppers, red chili peppers, parsley, watercress, and cantaloupe.
- *Beta-carotene:* Parsley, carrots, winter squash, sweet potatoes, yams, cantaloupe, apricots, spinach, kale, turnip greens, and citrus fruits.

An amino acid, beta-carotene belongs to a family of chemicals known as "carotenoids." People with a high level of beta-carotene in their blood have been found to have a lower risk not only of heart disease but also of cancer and stroke.

Your Three-Part Program for Heart Attack Prevention

4. Eat fish at least three times a week.
Eating fish will help protect your heart, because fish—particularly fatty fish, like salmon and mackerel—contain important omega-3 fatty acids. These substances, found only in fish, are heart protective. Since people sometimes overestimate the amount of fish they eat, you may supplement the omega-3 effect by taking fish oil tablets. In addition to helping prevent heart attacks, it was also thought that fish oil would help prevent potentially dangerous heart rhythm irregularities. Some research has cast doubt on that assumption, but fish oil is still considered generally healthy, especially for heart attack survivors.

5. Add fiber to your diet.
Fiber, the indigestible part of foods, is not absorbed into the bloodstream. In general, fiber is good to add to your diet, because it helps you feel full. There are two types of fiber; soluble and insoluble. Insoluble fiber passes through the body largely intact, and it is good for preventing constipation. Soluble fiber does this as well, but it also helps to lower cholesterol. Sources of soluble fiber include oat cereals, dried beans and peas, barley, flaxseed, oranges, apples, carrots, and psyllium husk, which is found in some fiber supplements.

6. Drink alcohol in moderation.
The moderate consumption of alcoholic beverages—be it wine, beer, or liquor—has been found to reduce the risk of heart disease. Evidence suggests much of this benefit comes from the fact that alcohol increases the amount of the "good" HDL cholesterol in the blood. There's also evidence that alcohol may favorably affect blood clotting, reducing heart attack risk. These protective effects are found no matter whether wine, beer, or liquor is consumed.

Chapter Ten

However, red wine and dark beer also may have antioxidant effects that can help retard the effects of aging on the heart's vessels. By the way, teetotalers can get this beneficial effect by drinking grape juice.

But, before you imbibe, there are other factors to take into account. First, the studies show that these protective effects are true only for those who indulge moderately. For women, this is defined as one drink, a standard drink being 12 ounces of beer, 4 ounces of wine, or 1.5 ounces of 80-proof spirit. Women who drink heavily are more prone to develop serious health problems, including high blood pressure, cardiomyopathy (a disease that weakens the heart muscle), and potentially deadly liver diseases like cirrhosis and hepatitis.

7. Take a daily multiple vitamin.
If you follow these dietary guidelines, you should get the recommended daily requirement of nutrients from the foods you eat. Sometimes, though, it's hard to be sure, so taking a multiple vitamin is a good dietary insurance policy. You don't need to waste your money on the supplements that fill supermarket and health shop shelves. There is currently insufficient evidence to recommend for or against the use of supplements for the prevention of heart disease. For instance, vitamin E, an antioxidant, was assumed for years to be cardio-protective. This has not been found to be the case, however. In fact, it's been repeatedly found that antioxidant supplements are not as beneficial as when the antioxidants are contained in whole foods.

Also, some supplements may do harm. Just because a supplement is sold in health food stores and labeled "natural" does not necessarily mean it's safe. Taking megadoses of some vitamins can be dangerous as well. Excessive amounts of vitamin D can interfere with calcium and phosphate levels in the body, and high doses of vitamin E can cause stomach upsets and abdominal pain or can interfere with the absorption of other fat soluble vitamins into the body.

There is, however, a lot of speculation about coenzyme Q10 (CoQ10), a fat-soluble, vitamin-like substance found in every human cell. It is involved in key biochemical reactions that produce energy in cells. It also acts like an antioxidant. It is found naturally in a variety of foods, including organ meats, such as heart, liver, and kidney, as well as in beef, soybean oil, sardines, mackerel, and peanuts. CoQ10 is also a very popular supplement sold to people who are seeking to protect the health of their heart. However, studies on people with angina and congestive heart failure have found conflicting results, so the American Heart Association doesn't recommend it.

Quitting smoking, exercising, and eating heart healthy—these are the three pillars of the plan that can help you prevent another heart attack. If you follow this program, you will not only prevent that heart attack, but you'll also feel better than you have in years.

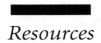

Resources

ORGANIZATIONS AND WEB SITES

Women's Health Hot Line
char@libov.com
www.libov.com

American Heart Association
731 Greenville Avenue
Dallas, TX 75231
800-227-2345
www.americanheart.org

National Heart, Lung, and Blood Institute (NHLBI) Information Center
P.O. Box 30105
Bethesda, MD 20824-0105
800-575-WELL
www.nhlbi.nih.gov

National Coalition for Women with Heart Disease (WomenHeart)
818 18th Street, NW
Suite 730
Washington, DC 20006
www.womenheart.org

Resources

Women's Heart Foundation
P.O. Box 7827
West Trenton, NJ 08628
Tel: 609-771-9600
Fax: 609-771-9427
www.womensheart.org
Tel: 202-728-7199
Fax: 202-728-7238

Black Women's Health Imperative
600 Pennsylvania Avenue, S.E.
Suite 310
Washington, DC 20003
Tel: 202-548-4000
Fax: 202-543-9743
www.blackwomenshealth.org

DASH Diet
www.nhlbi.nih.gov/health/public/heart/hbp/dash/

American Diabetes Association
1600 Duke Street
Alexandria, VA 11324
800-232-11324
www.diabetes.org

Harvard School of Public Health's Healthy Eating Pyramid (Mediterranean Diet)
www.hsph.harvard.edu/nutritionsource/pyramids.html

Resources

National High Blood Pressure Education Program
www.nhlbi.nih.gov/about/nhbpep/index.htm

National Cholesterol Education Program
www.nhlbi.nih.gov/chd/

Index

Index

Index

Index

Index

Index

Index

Index

Index

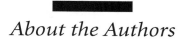

About the Authors

Harvey M. Kramer, M.D., is the director of Cardiovascular Disease Prevention at Praxair Regional Heart and Vascular Center at Danbury Hospital in Danbury, Connecticut. He is also assistant clinical professor of medicine at Yale University School of Medicine. He is a Fellow of the American College of Physicians and the American College of Cardiology and has been designated a specialist in Clinical Hypertension by the American Society of Hypertension. He is actively involved with the American Heart Association and formerly was president of the Connecticut American Heart Association.

Charlotte Libov is an award-winning medical author and contributor to the *New York Times* and other national publications. She has also written, produced, and appeared on programs for public television. Since undergoing open-heart surgery, she has become a popular speaker on women's health issues and is the founder of National Women's Heart Health Day. Her Web address is www.libov.com.